DEPARTMENT OF HEALTH

Report of the
Chief Medical Officer's Expert Group on
The Sleeping Position of Infants and Cot Death

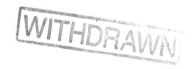

London : HMSO

618.92026 GRE

ISBN 0 11 321605 X

Contents

Part 1. The Report

Part 2.   The Evidence

Annexes

Glossary

I. The Report

1. *Introduction*

1.1   Cot death - the sudden, unexpected, and unexplained death of an infant - is not a new phenomenon: it has been known since biblical times ["And when I rose in the morning to give my child suck, behold, it was dead....." (1 Kings 3:21. King James Version)]. It is generally accepted that cot death does not have a single cause, but is one consequence of the interplay between factors that confer vulnerabilities upon a developing infant, and various external influences. This can result in a failure of breathing and circulation, and end in death. So far, *epidemiological* studies have made the largest contribution to our understanding of cot death. Such studies can rarely explain the events which lead to a particular outcome; but they can yield insights from which more discerning studies - including *intervention studies* - can begin.

1.2   Reports of epidemiological studies from several different countries have drawn renewed attention to particular *risk factors* in cot death. Those risk factors are laying infants to sleep on their fronts (prone), parental smoking, and inadvertent overheating. All are amenable to change. Therefore a number of programmes have been set up with the aim of influencing these factors and observing the effects. During 1991 there were preliminary reports of intervention programmes which had been conducted in Avon, England, and in New Zealand. They showed that a reduction in the proportion of infants sleeping on the front had been matched by a fall in the *incidence* of cot death.

1.3   The Chief Medical Officer therefore established this group to examine the findings, together with evidence from other studies, and to give advice.

Technical terms which are shown *in italics* appear in the Glossary

Terms of reference

1.4   Our initial terms of reference were:

"to consider the evidence relating to the sleeping position of infants and the risk of sudden infant death (cot death), and to advise the Chief Medical Officer".

We were also invited to extend our remit to consider other factors which were associated with cot death and which might also be amenable to intervention. During our deliberations, therefore, we examined published evidence on parental smoking, the thermal environment of infants, and breast-feeding.

Method of working

1.5   The group met for the first time on 29 October 1991 and met six times. On the basis of the evidence made available at the first meeting, including some not then published, we were able to arrive at a number of conclusions which formed the basis of our initial advice to the Chief Medical Officer, and upon which action quickly followed[1]. At subsequent meetings we considered further evidence that became available, together with published evidence on the additional factors that lay within our extended remit. We also addressed the need to monitor the effects of any new interventions that were introduced as a consequence of our advice.

Death in infancy

1.6   Today, in the United Kingdom, all but 8 out of every 1,000 liveborn infants survive to their first birthday. Among those who do not survive, the majority die because they are born too small, many of them being very premature; or because of a lethal malformation which is present at birth; or because of an overwhelming infection[2]. A few die from cancer or one of the rare, untreatable, degenerative diseases. But some infants die suddenly and unexpectedly, and even with careful investigation a sufficient cause cannot be found. These sudden, unexpected and unexplained infant deaths, are known as cot deaths or sudden infant deaths. 93% of these deaths occur during the *postneonatal* period (from 28 days of age up to 1 year) and constitute almost half of all postneonatal deaths. About 6% of sudden unexpected infant deaths occur earlier, during the *neonatal* period (at up to 28 days), and a very few after 1 year[3a, b].

1.7   In 1971 the terms cot death, sudden infant death, Sudden Infant Death Syndrome (SIDS) or similar term, became registrable as a cause of death. Since that time there has been evidence of a shift in certification practice, deaths being attributed to sudden infant death that previously might have been attributed to respiratory conditions. The *infant mortality rate* (deaths up to 1 year per 1,000 live births) attributed to sudden infant death rose steadily to 2.13 per 1,000 livebirths in 1982. There was a slight fall to 1.95 in 1984 and a rise to 2.30 in 1988. Since 1988 there has been a continual fall, to 1.70 and 1.44 per 1,000 livebirths in 1990 and 1991 respectively[3a, b].

1.8   The *postneonatal mortality rate* attributed to sudden infant death or respiratory conditions remained relatively constant until 1988; but since that time deaths attributed to either cause have fallen (Table 1, Fig 1). During the years 1988-1991 sudden infant deaths accounted for 2.01, 1.69, 1.48 and 1.25 postneonatal deaths per 1,000 livebirths. During the same period deaths due to respiratory disorders have fallen from 0.46 to 0.29 per 1,000 livebirths and those due to *congenital anomalies* from 0.59 to 0.50 per 1,000 livebirths. Postneonatal mortality overall has fallen from 4.11 per 1,000 livebirths in 1988 to 3.01 per 1,000 livebirths in 1991[3a,b].

1.9   Since 1988 a fall in the sudden infant death rate has also been seen in Scotland[4].

Nomenclature

1.10   Recently there have been discussions and correspondence over what precisely is meant by cot death (see Annex F). It has been recommended that the term "sudden infant death" should cover all infant deaths where "cot death","Sudden Infant Death Syndrome" or a similar term is included on the death

Table 1.   **Cumulative postneonatal deaths by selected causes, England and Wales, 1963-91.**

Rates per 1,000 livebirths of postneonatal deaths by selected causes 1963-91.

	1963	1964	1965	1966	1967	1968	1969	1970	1971	1972
SIDS						0	0	.06	.29	.60
+ Respiratory conditions	3.25	2.58	2.64	2.75	2.69	2.7	2.77	2.73	2.87	2.78
+ Congenital anomalies	4.72	3.98	3.95	4.01	3.84	3.98	3.97	3.97	4.09	3.97
+ Perinatal conditions	4.82	4.06	4.04	4.1	3.94	4.04	4.03	4.02	4.16	4.03
+ Injury and poisoning	5.39	4.71	4.71	4.74	4.54	4.65	4.7	4.57	4.64	4.46
+ Other conditions =	6.87	6.09	6.02	6.14	5.81	5.93	6.01	5.87	5.88	5.68
Total postneonatal										

	1973	1974	1975	1976	1977	1978	1979	1980	1981	1982
SIDS	.78	.85	.96	.96	1.08	1.13	1.27	1.44	1.55	1.73
+ Respiratory conditions	2.77	2.64	2.56	2.41	2.38	2.42	2.52	2.48	2.43	2.61
+ Congenital anomalies	3.99	3.78	3.63	3.37	3.37	3.35	3.37	3.31	3.33	3.54
+ Perinatal conditions	4.07	3.86	3.69	3.48	3.45	3.42	3.53	3.48	3.52	3.72
+ Injury and poisoning	4.5	4.24	4.03	3.83	3.75	3.71	3.85	3.7	3.74	3.91
+ Other conditions =	5.74	5.3	5.00	4.57	4.50	4.52	4.58	4.38	4.41	4.55
Total postneonatal										

	1983	1984	1985	1986	1987	1988	1989	1990	1991
SIDS	1.65	1.6	1.69	1.96	1.97	2.01	1.69	1.48	1.25
+ Respiratory conditions	2.36	3.15	2.27	2.43	2.40	2.57	2.03	1.78	1.54
+ Congenital anomalies	3.22	2.96	3.00	3.17	3.12	3.06	2.67	2.30	2.04
+ Perinatal conditions	3.47	3.19	3.24	3.48	3.37	3.38	2.97	2.62	2.35
+ Injury and poisoning	3.62	3.35	3.39	3.64	3.50	3.54	3.10	2.75	2.48
+ Other conditions =	4.29	3.91	3.98	4.28	4.14	4.11	3.69	3.32	3.01
Total postneonatal									

Source: OPCS

6

Fig 1. Cumulative postneonatal deaths by selected causes, England and Wales, 1963-1991

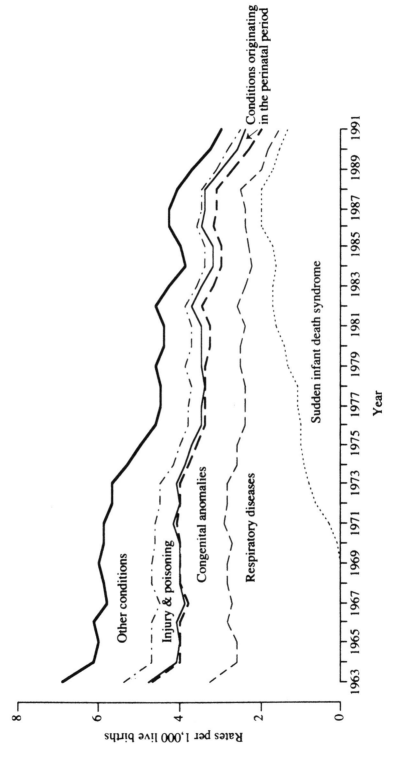

certificate, even when other conditions are also given. The term "Sudden Infant Death Syndrome" (SIDS, ICD 9th revision 798.0) should properly be confined to those cases where it is the only cause given for an infant death. However, the term is used more widely in some presentations of data. Since 1971 The Office of Population Censuses and Surveys (OPCS) has identified all infant deaths where the death certificate included the term cot death, sudden infant death or similar term. Subsequently, deaths which have another explanation are recoded, and those that remain are coded as Sudden Infant Death Syndrome (ICD 798.0). The figures given at 1.7 and 1.8 are taken from Office of Population Censuses and Surveys Mortality Statistics, Series DH3[3a,b]. They refer to the wider definition of sudden infant death.

Sudden Infant Death Syndrome (SIDS)

1.11   This term was coined in 1969 by a group in Seattle[5] and was defined as:

> "the sudden death of an infant or young child, which is unexpected by history, and in which a thorough postmortem examination fails to demonstrate an adequate cause of death".

It is a diagnosis of exclusion. The characteristic features are that with few exceptions it occurs in the first year of life (most often during the period 1 - 4 months), and is sudden, unexpected and unexplained. Deaths attributed to SIDS constitute the great majority of cot deaths (or deaths described by a similar term, such as "sudden infant death", "sudden, unexpected infant death", and its variants). We favour the term "cot death", which we have used throughout Part 1 of this Report as being synonymous with Sudden Infant Death Syndrome.

1.12   It has been remarked that if the sudden unexpected deaths of infants are subjected to thorough investigation, a probable cause of death will be found in a small proportion[6,7]. Such deaths are commonly due to overwhelming infection, or major unrecognised malformations, some of which are treatable. For these reasons parents should be encouraged to seek medical advice promptly if an infant is unwell or thought to be unwell.

8

It should, however, be emphasised that the majority of babies who succumb to cot death have not been significantly unwell in the preceding day or two[7].

Characteristics of cot death

1.13   Epidemiological studies from many parts of the world have shown a number of consistent features of cot death and have yielded considerable knowledge of the circumstances in which cot death occurs. Importantly, they have defined factors whose presence increases the risk. Studies published up to 1984 have been described and examined in detail in the monograph by Golding, Limerick and Macfarlane[8].

1.14   In brief, there is a typical age distribution for cot death, with a peak at 8-17 weeks of age. About 6% of these deaths occur during the first month of life. More boys are affected than girls. Cot death is more likely to occur in winter; the risk is increased in social classes IV and V; to the infants of young mothers; to infants with a large number of other siblings; and when only a short interval followed the previous pregnancy. The risk is greater if the child is one of a multiple birth, is preterm or of low birthweight.

Recent findings

1.15   Recently much attention has been given to findings that sleeping on the front (prone) is significantly more common among infants who die of cot death than among controls. There has also been an increasing emphasis on the risks associated with smoking by the mother or her partner during pregnancy and afterwards; and there is evidence that factors relating to the capacity of infants to control their temperature and the risk of overheating are also important. Non-breast-feeding has also been suggested as a risk factor for cot death, but the evidence is not consistent.

1.16   The published evidence is reviewed in Part 2 of this Report. It has not revealed an underlying cause of cot death, but it does point to factors in infant care that can be changed, with the expectation that the risk of cot death will be reduced.

Sleeping position of infants

1.17   We are aware of no evidence that babies in this country slept in
          other positions than on their backs (supine) until the beginning
          of this century, when the practice of laying infants on their sides
          began[9]. The side (lateral) position was adopted to avoid a stated
          danger of inhaling vomit, but the evidence on which this advice
          was based has not been found. This position was favoured until
          the late 1940s and 1950s, and possibly later. In 1961 there was a
          reference *(loc. cit.)* to placing babies on their fronts (prone) to
          reduce the risk of inhaling vomit. During the late 1960s and the
          1970s in special care baby units for vulnerable or sick infants,
          many of whom were premature, it became the practice to nurse
          infants on their fronts. This was based on physiological studies
          which showed that in these infants oxygenation was more
          efficient in the prone position[10]. Gradually the practice was
          adopted more generally, although there is no evidence that
          mature and older infants benefit in the same way.

1.18   There is evidence that practices have differed over time
          between countries of European heritage, and also between
          those countries and others, and between different cultural
          groups within them. It is unlikely that adequate information is
          available to document these changes fully, but data extracted by
          Beal and Finch from *retrospective case-control studies* are given in
          Table 2.

Sleeping position and cot death.

1.19   Evidence of a relationship between sleeping position and cot
          death had, until recently, come only from retrospective studies.
          Different definitions and methods have impeded comparisons
          between the studies and have hindered their acceptance[11].
          However, the consistency of a growing number of reports has
          caused increasing attention to be given to the sleeping position
          of infants as a factor, or proxy for some other factor, in cot
          death. Reports of the sequelae of interventions designed to
          change infant care practices, notably infant sleeping position
          have been especially persuasive, though not conclusive. They
          have now been followed by reports of four prospective

Table 2: **Sleeping position of control infants in retrospective case-control studies which examined the relationship between prone sleeping position and SIDS**

Place of study	Study period	Controls Total (n)	Prone (%)
South Australia	1980-84	156	38
South Australia	1985-89	182	29
France	Not stated	211	34
Melbourne, Australia	1980-82	393	41
The Netherlands	1980-86	320	62
Tasmania, Australia	1988-90	79	37
The Netherlands	1988	567	62
Avon/Somerset, UK	1987-89	134	57
Northern Ireland	1965-67	148	4
Belgium and France	1977-82	177	68
Hong Kong	1986-87	32	6
Tasmania, Australia	1980-86	329	43
Auckland, New Zealand	1987-88	503	43
Dunedin, New Zealand	1986-87	4041	42
UK	1976-79	273	25
Cologne, Germany	1974-84	306	40
Rennes, France	1984-85	318	30
Auckland, New Zealand	1970-82	1882	30
Avon, UK	1989-90	56	29

Source: Beal SM, Finch CF. An overview of retrospective case-control studies investigating the relationship between prone sleeping position and SIDS. J Paediatr Child Health 1991; 27: 334-339.

intervention studies although so far only two have been published in full[32,33].

Retrospective studies.

1.20   The first quantitative study of sleeping position in relation to cot death was by Adelson and Kinner in 1956[12]. They found that 65 out of 99 infants died whilst on their backs; but there were no data on the general *prevalence* of babies lying on their fronts in the population studied.

1.21   In 1965 Carpenter and Shadwick[13]. compared 110 cases of cot death with 110 controls, and found more cases than *controls* were on their fronts. This difference was *significant*[14].

1.22   Froggatt (1970)[15] reported that in the Northern Ireland population studies 7% of cases of cot death were usually placed on their fronts compared with 4% of controls, and 11% were usually placed on their backs compared with 34% of controls. He also observed that there was no significant difference between the usual sleeping position of the infant reported by parents and the position in which the infant was found after death.

1.23   Davies (1985)[16] found that cot death was rare in Hong Kong, where there was a cultural preference for placing infants on their backs. There were, however, no control subjects in the study.

1.24   A study which did not come to the attention of the English speaking world until 1990 was published in a German *Festschrift* in 1985[17]. 81% of cot death victims were found on their fronts compared with 40% of controls.

1.25   There were further studies during 1985-88. Beal[18] compared risk factors for cot death in relation to sudden infant death rates among different communities. She reported differences in the incidence of cot death according to the cultural practice of sleep positioning. The rate was lowest among South Sea Islanders, who almost invariably place infants on their backs; highest among Maoris, whose infants sleep on their fronts; and intermediate among infants of European descent, who were

12

mostly placed on their fronts. Beal recommended that putting infants to sleep on their fronts be avoided. Other studies from Australia[19,20], New Zealand[21], France[22], Holland[23] and England[24] also reported that more cot death victims were found on their fronts compared with controls.

1.26   Retrospective case-control studies from New Zealand[25] and Hong Kong[26] were published in 1989. In the former, 81% of cot death victims slept on their fronts compared with 49% of an *unmatched control* group. In the Hong Kong study 44% of cot death victims were found lying on their fronts compared with 7% of controls. A retrospective case-control study from Avon, England published in 1990[27] reported that cot death victims were more likely to have been sleeping on their fronts than were those in the control group. Lastly, in 1991, results from the first year of the New Zealand cot death study were published[28]. In addition to confirming many known risk factors for cot death the study identified three risk factors which were potentially amenable to change. They were the prone sleeping position of infants, maternal smoking and non-breast-feeding. These variables appeared to act independently.

Post-intervention studies

1.27   In 1988 Beal[29] reported a 30% reduction in the numbers of babies sleeping on their fronts in South Australia, and this change was associated with a fall of over 50% in the incidence of cot death. But the fall was not sustained.

1.28   After an influential lecture a public campaign began in the Netherlands in 1972, advising against laying infants to sleep on their backs. A detailed review of these events and their sequelae is given in the monograph by Engelberts[30]. Before 1971 the incidence of cot death in the Netherlands was very low - 0.46 per 1,000 livebirths. Following the new advice it rose to 1.3 per 1,000 livebirths.

1.29   In 1987 a new public campaign was mounted in the Netherlands to reverse the practice, by advising against laying infants on their fronts. Engelberts and De Jonge[31] subsequently reported a fall of 40% in the incidence of cot death in 1988 compared with the previous year.

Prospective studies

1.30   A single *prospective study* from Tasmania, Australia, by Dwyer et al[32] had been published when we began our deliberations. This was a cohort study of 4,103 infants who had been assessed at birth as being at high risk. 29 died of cot death. A *matched* analysis, which controlled for birthweight and maternal age, showed that after correction for these *confounding variables* there was an increased risk of cot death for infants who were sleeping on their fronts at one month.

1.31   The Avon retrospective case-control study led to a local awareness campaign which began in late 1989. A subsequent study with two groups of controls - matched and randomly enroled - showed falls in the proportion of infants sleeping on their fronts in both control groups. There was a fall in the incidence of cot death close to that predicted from the initial study. These findings were made available to us during our deliberations and have now been published[33].

1.32   Similar campaigns in Australia and New Zealand have been followed by falls in the incidence of cot death, although data on infant sleeping positions before and after these interventions have yet to be published in full[34,35].

Conclusions: sleeping position and cot death

1.33   These studies are consistent in showing an increased risk of cot death when infants are on their fronts compared with other positions. In the retrospective studies *odds ratios* were in the range 1.9-12.7; in the post-intervention study[33] it was 9.1; and in the prospective study[32] now published it was 4.5 (see Part 2; 1: Table 1).

1.34   In the intervention studies described, falls in the proportion of infants placed on their fronts were consistently associated with falls in the incidence of cot death.

1.35   Not all infants who suffer cot death are found lying on their fronts; neither do the great majority of infants who sleep on their fronts die of cot death. Therefore sleeping on the front is not a sufficient cause of cot death.

On the side or on the back?

1.36 Most studies have compared lying on the front with other positions, without discriminating between the side and the back positions. Mitchell[35] reported an unpublished analysis of the data of the New Zealand study which suggested that side sleeping was associated with a *relative risk* of 2.0, and sleeping on the front with a relative risk of 6.7, compared with sleeping on the back. In the Netherlands, Engelberts[30] found that the relative risk of always being placed on the front was greater than that of sometimes being placed on the front, which was greater than the risk of being placed on the back or on the side. It was reported from Avon that most infants who rolled over after being laid to sleep on their sides, rolled on to the back[36]. On the other hand, 6 (18%) of those who died had rolled on to the front from the side position[66].

Concerns

1.37 We have noted (1.17) the concern to avoid the possible risk of inhaling vomit. In many societies the majority of infants sleep on the back and there is no evidence of an increased risk of death in normal infants from aspiration or choking. There has also been concern about infants who are being treated in splints (eg von Rosen splints) for congenital dislocation of the hip, and the risk of laying them on the back for sleep. There is no published evidence that this is more hazardous. In the Avon studies there were cot deaths among such infants when they were sleeping on the front.

Exceptions

Some infants are at particular risk of airway obstruction (notably those with *Pierre-Robin syndrome*) and should be nursed on the front. There might be a temporary advantage for newborn infants with breathing problems from sleeping on the front. In infants with severe *gastro-oesophageal reflux* there might be some benefit from sleeping on the front which must be weighed carefully against the increased risk of cot death. Newborn infants who find difficulty clearing airway secretions might benefit from the side sleeping position for the first few days.

Smoking and cot death

1.39   The harmful effects of smoking upon the unborn child have been recognised since 1957. Many studies have shown that exposure to smoking during pregnancy is an important risk factor in fetal and neonatal death[36]. Maternal smoking during pregnancy, and the exposure of an infant to paternal smoking has adverse effects upon infancy and childhood, including impaired growth and development. An association of cot death with passive smoking was first reported in 1976[37], and with smoking during pregnancy in 1979[38].

1.40   Five prospective *cohort studies*[38-42] and numerous retrospective case-control studies [26,28,37,43-50] have shown a strong, consistent relationship between maternal smoking and the risk of cot death. Moreover, the risk increases with the numbers of cigarettes smoked. There is evidence that passive smoking might also make a significant contribution[50]. The separate contributions to the risk of cot death from maternal smoking in pregnancy, passive smoking in pregnancy and passive smoking in infancy have not yet been determined.

Conclusions: smoking and cot death

1.41   The risk of cot death is increased when an infant is exposed to cigarette smoke during the period before birth and afterwards. There is an increased risk with both maternal and paternal smoking, and the risk is related to the number of cigarettes smoked daily. The odds ratios are usually at least 2 and are as high as 4.8 in heavy smokers[41,50].

1.42   These findings, which are described fully in Part 2, provide the basis for clear advice against exposing infants to the effects of cigarette smoke, both before birth and during infancy.

Thermal environment and cot death

1.43   Until recently the thermal environment of infants had been given less attention than sleeping position, and the body of scientific evidence is small. Extreme cold or extreme heat can cause the death of an infant, but in such circumstances the cause is usually clear. Surroundings that are less obviously extreme might cause, or be a contributing factor in cot death[27,51,52]. The evidence is considered in Part 2 of the Report.

1.44   A matched case-control study in Avon[27] showed that an increased risk of cot death was associated with either or both of two factors which might lead to overheating. They were the insulation provided by bedding and clothing, and room heating. A study in Tasmania[53] showed similar results.

1.45   Although high insulation has been shown to be a risk factor for cot death, there is evidence that infants in normal circumstances can tolerate a wide range of insulation, and it seems unlikely that high insulation alone is a cause of cot death[27,51-57]. However, there is evidence that it might interact adversely with other factors (loc. cit.), namely:

> the temperature of the baby's environment
> direct heating
> covering the head, with bedding or a hat
> sleeping on the front
> fever as a result of infection.

1.46   The Avon studies[27,56] showed that:

> room heating had been on all night for a significantly higher proportion of cot death victims than controls

> cot death victims with viral infections had significantly higher insulation than controls

> there was a greater risk of cot death among infants sleeping on their fronts if they were heavily insulated

> 25% of cot death victims were found with their heads covered by bedding or a hat, compared with none among controls.

Conclusions: Thermal environment and cot death

1.47   Inadvertent overheating, to which various factors might contribute, probably increases the risk of cot death.

1.48   This finding, together with other observations described in Part

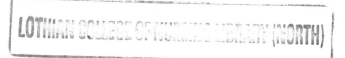

2, allow balanced advice to be given to parents, with the possibility for further reducing the risk of cot death.

Breast-feeding and cot death

1.49   There is no consistent evidence as yet on breast-feeding and cot death. Maternal smoking influences breast-feeding: mothers who smoke during pregnancy are not only less likely to start breast-feeding, but having started they are more likely to stop early[67]. Unfortunately, very few studies of breast-feeding and cot death have taken account of smoking, itself a significant factor in cot death. The evidence is given in Part 2.

Conclusions: breast-feeding and cot death

1.50   Whilst breast-feeding has many benefits and few disadvantages, it is not evident from published studies that breast-feeding reduces the risk of cot death.

Other aspects of infant care and cot death

1.51   We recognise that other aspects of infant care might be important in cot death although the evidence is largely descriptive. For example, it has been pointed out that putting infants on their own to sleep, a common practice in Western countries, has few historical or cultural precedents[9,58,59]. Some communities, both in this country and elsewhere in the world, where babies sleep close to their parents, are also those in which it is customary to lay infants to sleep on their backs. Careful studies would be required to appraise these influences.

1.52   If the sudden unexpected deaths of infants are subjected to thorough investigation a treatable cause of death is found in a small proportion of them[6,7]. For these reasons parents and others who are entrusted with the care of an infant should be encouraged to seek medical advice promptly if the infant is unwell or thought to be unwell (see 1.12).

Conclusions

1.53   The evidence on which our conclusions and recommendations are based is presented and discussed more fully in Part 2 of the Report. Some of the evidence was not available to us when we gave our initial advice; but we have found no reason to modify our views except in detail and emphasis.

1.54   First, we **affirm** our view that the risk of cot death can be reduced if babies are not placed on their fronts when they are laid down to sleep. We now **conclude** that the risk can be further reduced if (with the exceptions described at 1.38, and on medical advice) babies are laid on their backs rather than on their sides (see 1.36). We also **affirm** that there is no published evidence of an increased risk of death in normal infants from aspiration or choking.

1.55   Secondly, we **emphasise** that the risk of cot death is increased when an infant is exposed to cigarette smoke during the period before birth and afterwards. The risk is increased when the mother smokes and when the father smokes. Smoking might have effects before birth or during infancy, although the data are insufficient to quantify the separate risks. Similarly, there are inadequate data on the effects of others smoking near the baby. We **conclude** that the increased risk overall when an infant has been exposed to smoking could, with heavy smokers, be close to that associated with laying a baby on the front to sleep.

1.56   Thirdly, although we are able to give only general advice on reducing the risks associated with overwrapping or overheating a baby, we wish to **emphasise** the particular hazard of overheating when a baby is feverish or unwell. There are insufficient data to quantify these risks, but they may be substantial.

1.57   There is evidence that some of these risks might be interactive, notably those associated with overheating and overwrapping, infection, and sleeping position.

1.58   We **conclude** that the risks of cot death are increased:

       (i)   when an infant is laid down to sleep on the front (except in particular circumstances, on medical advice)

Risk increased 3 to 8 fold

and also that the risk is least when an infant is laid on the back to sleep (except in the circumstances described).

(ii)   when an infant is exposed to cigarette smoke during the period before birth and afterwards. The risk is increased when the mother smokes and when the father smokes. The risk is related to the numbers of cigarettes smoked, and overall

Risk increased 2-3 fold or more

(iii)   when an infant is overwrapped or overheated, especially if feverish or unwell

Risk increased (substantially)
(but not yet quantified).

Recommendations

1.59   We **recommend** that:-

Infants should not be laid to sleep on their fronts (except in particular circumstances, on medical advice) and the great majority of infants should be nursed on their backs.

If the side position is chosen, the lower arm should be well in front of the body so that the infant does not roll on to the front. We do not recommend placing devices such as wedges and rolled up sheets behind the infant: because doing so might increase the risk of rolling on to the front.

Concerns

We have noted the concern to avoid the possible risk of inhaling vomit. In many societies the majority of infants sleep on the back and there is no evidence of an increased risk of death in normal infants from aspiration or choking.

Exceptions

Some infants are at particular risk of airway obstruction (notably those with Pierre-Robin syndrome) and should be nursed on the front. There might be a temporary advantage for newborn infants with breathing problems from sleeping on the front. In infants with severe gastro-oesophageal reflux there might be some benefit from sleeping on the front which must be weighed carefully against the increased risk of cot death. Newborn infants who find difficulty clearing airway secretions might benefit from the side sleeping position for the first few days.

Infants should not be exposed to cigarette smoke either before birth or afterwards.

The risk of cot death is increased, both with maternal and paternal smoking. The separate effects before birth and afterwards are not known. However, the risk is related to the numbers of cigarettes smoked, and overall are increased 2-3 fold or more.

Infants should not be overwrapped or overheated, especially when they are feverish or unwell.

Guidance available to parents and others who have responsibilities for the care of infants should incorporate the following points:

- the room where an infant sleeps should be t a temperature which is comfortable for lightly clothed adults, ie 16-20°C;
- indoors, infants need little more bedding than adults;
- bedding should not be excessive for the temperature of the room;
- bedding should be arranged so that the infant is unlikely to slip underneath; for example, it can be made up so that the infant's feet come down to the end of the cot;
- duvets should not be used for infants under one year;
- bedding should not be increased when the infant is unwell or feverish;
- whilst asleep an infant should not be exposed to direct heating; for example, from a hot water bottle, electric blanket, or radiant heater;
- an infant over one month, at home, does not need to be kept as warm as in the hospital nursery;
- an infant over one month should not wear hats indoors for sleeping unless the room is very cold.

But when infants are taken outdoors in cold weather they must be adequately wrapped.

Breast-feeding should be encouraged wherever possible. It has many benefits and few disadvantages, although the evidence from published studies does not consistently show that breast-feeding affects the risk of cot death.

Parents, and others who are entrusted with the care of infants, should be encouraged to seek medical advice promptly if an infant is unwell or thought to be unwell.

A small proportion of the sudden unexpected deaths of infants are due to overwhelming infection or major unrecognised malformations, some of which are treatable. For these reasons parents should be encouraged to seek medical advice promptly if an infant is unwell or thought to be unwell. It should , however, be emphasised that the majority of babies who succumb to cot death have not been significantly unwell in the preceding day or two.

Public awareness programmes

1.60   We have referred to the recommendation by Beal that putting infants to sleep on their fronts be avoided (see 1.25) and the sequel to this advice (1.27). Subsequently, on the basis of the retrospective studies reported from Australia, New Zealand, Holland, and Avon in England, public awareness programmes were undertaken in attempts to reduce mortality from cot death. In Holland the reported association between sleeping position and cot death led in October 1987 to an official policy recommending that parents should not put their babies down to sleep on the front. In March 1991 the New Zealand National Cot Death Prevention Programme was begun. The Programme was aimed to change three aspects of infant care, namely, sleeping on the front, maternal smoking and not breast-feeding. A local programme similar to that in New Zealand had been instituted in Avon in 1990, with advice on sleeping position, thermal care of infants, illness management of infants and parental smoking. The advice encouraged breast-feeding for its known benefits but was careful to point out that lack of breast-feeding had not been shown to be a risk factor in Avon.

1.61   A national professional and public education programme which reflected our initial advice was begun in England and Wales, and in Scotland and Northern Ireland in October 1991[1]. It is outlined in the Annexes to our Report. Similar advice has now been given by the American Academy of Pediatrics [60,61], and by the Canadian Paediatric Society/Societe canadienne de pediatrie[62].

Consequences of public awareness programmes

1.62   If the associations between laying a baby to sleep on the front, cigarette smoking, overheating, non-breast-feeding (and other infant care practices) and cot death were not merely proxies for other, more direct (*causal*) influences, changes in these practices should be matched by changes in the incidence of cot death. There are now several published reports of studies to assess the effects of programmes designed to bring about such changes. They have provided convincing evidence that when those who are entrusted with the care of babies and infants take a number of simple precautions, the risks of cot death can be reduced. A reduction in the prevalence of sleeping on the front has been accompanied by a fall in the incidence of cot death[30-33]. The studies reported have not, so far, enabled conclusions to be drawn in relation to changes in exposure to smoking or in the thermal environment of infants.

1.63   The incidence of cot death in England and Wales following the national campaign has shown a dramatic fall (Table 3, Fig 2).

1.64   It is not claimed that removal of these hazards will eliminate cot death – that will not be possible until the underlying causes and the processes which lead to death are better understood – but it will reduce the risk.

1.65   By far the majority of babies who are laid on their fronts to sleep do not succumb to cot death; and neither are all babies who sleep on their backs spared. The majority of babies who are exposed to cigarette smoke do not die; nor do the great majority of babies who are feverish or unwell. But in every instance – by taking precautions that we advise – it is possible to reduce the risk.

Monitoring the consequences of interventions

1.66   Studies of specified public interventions in this area of infant care have four kinds of purpose, and all are important in order to guide future action. They are:

(i)   To assess the effectiveness of the national education campaign ("Back to Sleep") in reaching and being understood by health professionals and the public.

(ii)   To assess changes in infant care practice in respect of sleeping position, exposure to smoking, thermal care, illness management and breast-feeding; and whether they are sustained.

(iii)   To determine whether the changes observed are associated with the predicted changes in the incidence of cot death.

Table 3 **SIDS DEATHS (ICD 798.0)** England and Wales. Quarterly figures

Quarter	1989	1990	1991	*1992
March	406	365	321	128
June	238	255	252	110
September	192	176	150	86
December	354	283	189	143

Data: OPCS   *Provisional

Fig 2   Sudden Infant Death Syndrome (ICD 798.0) England and Wales.
Quarterly figures (Deaths at 28 days and over).

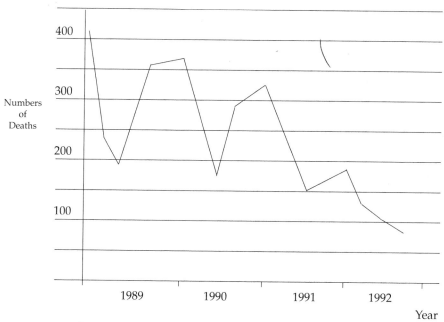

Data: OPCS (see Table 3)

25

(iv)   To determine whether those changes have significant inadvertent consequences, particularly a shift in the pattern of infant morality by cause and over time, or significant non-fatal consequences for infants, or for the parents and others who are entrusted with their care.

1.67   We **recommend** that the Department of Health continues to encourage and support programmes to monitor the effectiveness of the "Back to Sleep" campaign, and the consequences.

1.68   The Department of Health has already taken steps to follow up the advice given by the Chief Medical Officer[1] and the "Back to Sleep" campaign begun in 1991. They include:

(i)   Commissioning surveys to determine public awareness and understanding of the messages of the campaign, in the aftermath and subsequently (see Annex G).

(ii)   Reinforcing the importance of the "Back to Sleep" campaign and the Confidential Enquiry into Stillbirths and Deaths in Infancy, in Priorities and Planning Guidance for 1993-94 from the National Health Service (NHS) Management Executive[63].

(iii) Reinforcing NHS awareness of "Back to Sleep" before the onset of winter 1992-93, by means of an Executive Letter to health authorities and Trusts[64].

(iv)   Encouraging close cooperation with professional and voluntary bodies in this and further work, through the participation of their representatives on this Group and on the National Advisory Body which oversees and guides the Confidential Enquiry into Stillbirths and Deaths in Infancy [65].

(v)   Commissioning research through the NHS Research and Development programme, which also complements and strengthens that funded by other agencies; notably the Medical Research Council, The Foundation for the Study of Infant Deaths and the recently established Anne Diamond Cot Death Appeal.

(vi)   The Health Education Authority and the health education agencies in Scotland, Wales and Northern Ireland provide booklets which contain information on infant care. They are 'The Pregnancy Book', 'Birth to five', and 'Play it safe'. All contain up-to-date advice in relation to cot death and ways of reducing the risks (see Annex D).

(vii)   Commissioning analyses of data on infant care practice, collected by the Avon Longitudinal study of Pregnancy and Childbirth (ALSPAC) in Avon (see Annex H).

1.69   We **commend** these actions, and the alliances that have been developed.

Recommendations for further action

1.70   We **recommend** that there should be continuing review, to ensure that the benefits of applying the new knowledge to infant care are fully realised, together with monitoring and assessments of the kind described at 1.66.

1.71   We also **recommend** that in addition to any programmes that may be considered appropriate by the National Advisory Body for the Confidential Enquiry into Stillbirths and Deaths in Infancy, the Department of Health should encourage and support other necessary programmes to monitor those aspects described at 1.66 which are not covered elsewhere.

1.72   We **recommend** that our Report be brought to the notice of the Chief Executive, NHS Management Executive, with whom lies the operational responsibility for ensuring that services are managed and delivered with improved effectiveness.

Further research

1.73   From the research data available to us it is not to be expected that removal of the risk factors to which we have drawn attention will eliminate cot death. It is likely that there are other factors which cannot be influenced without additional knowledge. They might include anomalies of physical development that confer vulnerabilities upon the infant: physical and biological agents (including infectious agents); and social and cultural influences whose effects upon infants are poorly understood. It will, therefore, be necessary to continue biomedical and health service research into cot deaths, and other infant deaths of unknown cause.

1.74   We **recommend** that carefully designed and well-conducted studies be mounted into the antecedents and circumstances of unexplained infant deaths, the associated socio-biological factors, and the pathology of cot death, to learn more of known and possible risk factors, and their interplay.

1.75   We **recommend** that the attention of the Director of NHS Research and Development be drawn to these needs.

References

1.   Department of Health. *Sleeping position of infants and the risk of cot death (sudden infant death).* Heywood (Lancashire): Department of Health, 1991. (Professional letter: PL/CMO(91)16, PL(CNO) (91)11).

2.   Office of Population Censuses and Surveys. *Mortality Statistics: perinatal and infant: social and biological factors.* London: HMSO, 1978-90. (Series DH3).

3a.   Office of Population Censuses and Surveys. *Sudden infant death syndrome.* OPCS monitor series DH3. London: HMSO, 1980-90. (DH3 80/3 to 91/1).

3b.   Office of Population Censuses and Surveys. *Sudden infant deaths 1990-91.* OPCS monitor series DH3. London: HMSO, 1992. (DH3 92/2).

4.   Gibson A, Brooke H, Keeling J. Reduction in sudden infant death syndrome in Scotland. *Lancet* 1991; 338: 1595.

5.   Bergman AB, Beckwith JB, Ray CC. *Sudden infant death syndrome.* Seattle: University of Washington Press, 1970.

6.   Gilbert RE, Fleming PJ, Berry J, Rudd PT. Signs of illness preceding sudden unexpected death in infants. *BMJ* 1990; 301: 45-46.

7.   McLoughlin A. Sudden infant deaths in Tameside, *Health Visitor,* 1988; 61; 235-237.

8.   Golding J, Limerick S, Macfarlane A. *Sudden infant deaths. Patterns, puzzles and problems.* Somerset, England: Open Books Publishing Ltd, 1985.

9.   Hiley C. Babies' sleeping position. *BMJ* 1992; 305: 115.

10.   Martin RJ, Herrell N, Rubin D, Fanaroff A. Effect of supine and prone positions on arterial oxygen tension in the preterm infant. *Pediatrics* 1979; 63: 528-531.

11.   Beal SM, Finch C. An overview of retrospective case-control studies investigating the relationship between prone sleeping position and SIDS. J *Paediatric Child Health* 1991; 27: 334-339.

12. Adelson L, Kinney ER. Sudden and unexpected death in infancy and childhood. *Pediatrics* 1956; 17:663-697.

13. Carpenter RG, Shaddick CW. Role of infection, suffocation, and bottle-feeding in cot death. *Br J Prev Soc Med.* 1965; 19:1-7.

14. Beal SM. Sleeping position and SIDS. *Lancet.* 1988; 2: 512.

15. Froggatt P. *Epidemiological aspects of the Northern Ireland Study.* In: Bergman AB, Beckwith JB, Ray CG, eds. Proceedings of the second international conference on causes of sudden death in infants. Seattle: University of Washington Press; 1970: 34-46.

16. Davies DP. Cot death in Hong Kong: a rare problem? *Lancet.* 1985; 2: 1346-1349.

17. Saternus K-S. Plotzlicher *Kindstod: eine Folge der Bauchlage?* In: Festschrift Professor Leithoff. Heidelberg, Germany: Kriminalistik Verlag; 1985: 67-81.

18. Beal SM. Sudden infant death syndrome: epidemiological comparisons between South Australia and communities with a different incidence. *Aust Paediatr J* 1986; 22 (Suppl.): 13-16.

19. Cameron MH, Williams AL. Development and testing of scoring systems for predicting infants with high-risk of sudden infant death syndrome in Melbourne. *Aust Paediatr J* 1986; 22 (Suppl.): 37-45.

20. McGlashan ND. Sleeping position and SIDS. *Lancet* 1986; 1: 106.

21. Tonkin SL, Infant Mortality. Epidemiology of cot deaths in Auckland. *NZ Med J* 1986; 99: 924-926.

22. Senecal J. Roussey M, Defawe G, Delahaye M. Piquermal B. Procubitus et mort subite inattendue du norrisson. *Arch Fr Pediatr.* 1987; 44: 131-136.

23. DeJonge GA, Engelberts AC, Koomen-Liefting AJM, Kostense PJ. Cot death and prone sleeping position in the Netherlands. *BMJ* 1989; 298: 722.

24. Nicoll JP, O'Cathain A. Sleeping position and SIDS. *Lancet* 1988; ii: 106.

25.   Nelson EAS, Taylor BJ, Mackay SC. Child care practices and the sudden infant death syndrome. *Aust Paediatr J* 1989; J. 25: 202-204.

26.   Lee NYY, Chan YF, Davies DP, Lau E, Yip DCP. Sudden infant death syndrome in Hong Kong: confirmation of low incidence. *BMJ* 1989; 298: 721.

27.   Fleming PJ, Gilbert R, Azaz Y. et al. Interaction between bedding and sleeping position in the sudden infant death syndrome: a population-based case-control study. *BMJ* 1990; 301: 85-89.

28.   Mitchell EA, Scragg R, Stewart AW, Becroft DMO, Taylor BJ, Ford RPK, et al. Results from the first year of the New Zealand cot death study. *N Z Med J* 1991; 104: 71-76.

29.   Beal SM. Sleeping position and sudden infant death syndrome. *Med J Aust.* 1988: 149: 562.

30.   Engelberts AC. *Cot death in the Netherlands: An epidemiological study.* MD thesis, VU University Press, Amsterdam. 1991.

31.   Engelberts AC, DeJonge GA. Choice of sleeping position for infants: possible association with cot death. *Arch Dis Child* 1990; 65: 462-467.

32.   Dwyer T. Ponsonby A-LB, Newman NM, Gibbons LE. Prospective cohort study of prone sleeping position and sudden infant death syndrome. *Lancet* 1991; 337: 1244-1247.

33.   Wigfield RE, Fleming PJ, Berry PJ, Rudd PT, Golding J. Can the fall in Avon's sudden infant death rate be explained by changes in sleeping position? *BMJ* 1992; 304: 282-283.

34.   Mitchell EA, Engelberts AC. Sleeping position and cot deaths. *Lancet* 191; 338: 192.

35.   Mitchell EA. Cot death: Should the prone sleeping position be discouraged? *J. Paediatr Child Health* 1991; 27: 319-321.

36.   Golding J, Fleming PJ, Parkes S. Cot deaths and sleep position changes. *Lancet* 1992; 339: 748-749.

37.   Bergman AB, Wiesner LA. Relationship of passive cigarette

smoking to suden infant death syndrome. *Pediatrics* 1976; 58: 665-668.

38.   Lewark N, van den Berg BJ, Beckwith JB. Sudden infant death syndrome risk factors. *Clinical Pediatrics* 1979; 18: 405-11.

39.   Haglund B, Cnattimgius S. Cigarette smoking as a risk factor for sudden infant death syndrome: a population-based study. *American Journal of Public Health* 1990; 80: 29-32.

40.   Wierenga H. Brand R, Geudeke T, et al. Prenatal risk factors for cot death in very preterm and small-for-gestational-age infants. *Early Human Development* 1990; 23: 15-26.

41.   Murphy JF, Newcombe RG, Sibert JR. The epidemiology of sudden infant death syndrome. *J Epidem Common Health* 1982; 36: 17-21.

42.   Bulterys MG, Greenland S, Kraus JF. Chronic fetal hypoxia and sudden infant death syndrome: interaction between maternal smoking and low haematocrit during pregnancy. *Pediatrics* 1990; 86: 535-540.

43.   Rintahaka PJ, Hirvonen J. The epidemiology of sudden infant death syndrome in Finland 1969-1980. *Forensic Science International* 1986; 30: 219-233.

44.   McLoughlin A. Sudden infant deaths in Tameside. *Health Visitor* 1988; 61: 235-237.

45.   Gilbert R. Unpublished MD thesis.

46.   Hoffman HJ, Hunter JC, Ellish NJ, et al. *Adverse reproductive factors and the sudden infant death syndrome.* In: Harper RM, Hoffman HJ, (eds) Sudden Infant Death Syndrome. Risk factors and Basic Mechanisms. New York: PMA Publishing Corp, 1988; 153-175.

47.   Unsigned editorial. Choice of cases - with special reference to SIDS. *Pediatric & Perinatal Epidemiology* 1991; 5: 1-3.

48.   Malloy MH, Kleinman JC, Land GH, et al. The association of maternal smoking with age and cause of infant death. *American Journal of Epidemiology* 1988; 128: 46-55.

49.   McGlashan MD. Sudden infant deaths in Tasmania, 1980-1986: A 7 year prospective study. *Social Science and Medicine* 1989; 29: 1015-1026.

50.   Nicholl JP, O'Cathain A. *Antenatal smoking, postnatal passive smoking, and sudden infant death syndrome.* In: Effects of Smoking on the Fetus, Neonate and Child. Ed Poswillo D, Alberman E. Oxford: Oxford Medical Publications 1992.

51.   Bacon CJ, Bell SA, Clulow EE, et al. How mothers keep their babies warm. *Arch Dis Child* 1991; 66: 627-632.

52.   Fleming PJ, Azaz Y, Wigfield R, et al. *Laboratory and community studies of thermal balance in infants: possible relevance to SIDS.* Proc. 2nd SIDS Inernat Conf. Ed Walker A. Perinatology Press, New York 1992 (in press).

53.   Ponsonby A-L, Dwyer T, Gibbons LE, et al. Thermal environment and sudden infant death syndrome: case-conrol study. *BMJ* 1992; 304: 277-282.

54.   Anderson ES, Wailoo MP, Petersen SA. Use of thermographic imaging to study babies sleeping at home. *Arch Dis Child* 1990; 1266-67.

55.   Kerslake DMcK. The insulation provided by infant's bedclothes. *Ergonomics* 1991; 34: 893-907.

56.   Gilbert RE, Rudd PT, Berry PJ, et al. Combined effect of infection and heavy wrapping in sudden infant death. *Arch Dis Child* 1992; 67: 171-177.

57.   Nelson EAS, Taylor BJ, Weatherall IL, 1989. Sleeping position and infant bedding may predispose to hyperthermia and the sudden infant death syndrome. *Lancet* 1989; i: 199-201.

58.   Keeley D. Reducing the risks in the sudden infant death syndrome. *BMJ* 1992; 304: 775.

59.   Davies DP, Gantley M, Murcott A. Reducing the risks in sudden infant death syndrome. *BMJ* 1992; 304: 775.

60.   Kattwinkel J. Brooks J, Myerberg D. American Academy of Pediatrics Task Force on Infant Positioning and SIDS. *Pediatrics* 1992; 89: 1120-1126.

61.   Guntheroth WG, Spiers PS. Sleeping Prone and the Risk of Sudden Infant Death Syndrome. *JAMA* 1992; 267: 2359-2362.

62.   Canadian Paediatric Society / Societe' canadienne de pediatrie. Press release, September 12, 1992. Ottawa, Ontario, Canada.

63.   Department of Health. *Priorities and planning guidance for the NHS for 1993/94.* London: Department of Health, 1992. (Executive letter: EL(92)47).

64.   Department of Health. *"Back to Sleep" campaign and reducing the risk of cot death.* London: Department of Health, 1992. (Executive letter El(92)85).

65.   Department of Health. *Confidential enquiry into stillbirths and deaths in infancy (CESDI).* London: Department of Health, 1992. (Executive letter: EL(92)64).

66.   *Effects of Smoking on the Fetus, Neonate and Child.* Ed Poswillo D, Alberman E. Oxford: Oxford Medical Publications 1992.

67.   Office of Population Censuses and Surveys. *Infant feeding* 1990. London: HMSO, 1992.

2. *Summary of Evidence with Conclusions & Recommendations*

2.1 We were asked to consider the evidence relating to the sleeping position of infants and the risk of sudden infant death (cot death), and to advise the Chief Medical Officer. We were also invited to extend our remit to consider other factors that are associated with sudden infant death and might also be amenable to interventions. During our deliberations, therefore, we examined published evidence on parental smoking, the thermal environment of infants, and breast-feeding.

Sleeping position and cot death

2.2 Over 20 case-control studies from many countries have been published on the association between infant sleeping position and the risk of cot death. In all of these studies the risk was found to be higher for infants sleeping on their fronts (prone). Concerns about bias in the original retrospective studies have not been substantiated in a recent prospective study, which confirmed the increased risk associated with sleeping on the front. Preliminary reports of interventions which were aimed at changing infant sleeping practices have now been published. In all of these interventions a reduction in the prevalence of sleeping on the front was accompanied by a fall in the incidence of cot death. These findings suggest that the relationship is causal, sleeping on the front increasing the risk of cot death by 3-8 fold. Why this should be is unclear, but it may be related to airway obstruction, or heat stress to which an infant sleeping on the front might be subject. Evidence on the side sleeping position is inconclusive, but suggests that the risk is somewhat higher than it is for infants sleeping on the back, although lower than for infants sleeping on the front.

2.3 In many societies the majority of infants sleep on their backs and there is no evidence that normal infants are at increased risk of death by aspiration or choking in that position.

2.4 Some infants (eg those with Pierre-Robin syndrome) should be nursed on the front because of the particular risk of airway obstruction; for others (eg newborn infants with respiratory problems) there might be some temporary advantage from sleeping on the front; and for others (eg those with severe gastro-oesophageal reflux) there might be some benefits from sleeping on the front which must be carefully weighed against the increased risk of cot death. Some newborn infants experience difficulty in clearing airway secretions and might benefit from the side sleeping position for the first few days.

Conclusions

We **conclude** that the risk of cot death is increased when an infant is laid down to sleep on the front (except in particular circumstances, on medical advice).

Risk increased 3 to 8 fold

We also **conclude** that the risk is least when an infant is laid down to sleep on the back (except in the circumstances described above).

Recommendations

We **recommend** that, apart from the exceptions given above, the great majority of infants should be nursed on their backs.

If the side position is chosen, the lower arm should be well in front of the body so that the infant does not roll on to the front. Devices such as wedges and rolled up sheets placed behind the infant might increase the risk of rolling on to the front, and are **not recommended**.

Parental smoking and cot death

2.5   There have been five cohort studies in which information on maternal smoking was collected prospectively. All showed a strong and statistically significant relationship between maternal smoking and the risk of cot death. Moreover, the risk was dose dependent. Similar results have been obtained from case-control studies in which information was collected retrospectively. There is also evidence from three studies that passive smoking may be important. The separate contributions to the risk of cot death of maternal smoking in pregnancy, passive smoking in pregnancy, and passive smoking postnatally have not yet been determined.

Conclusions

We **conclude** that the risk of cot death is increased when an infant is exposed to cigarette smoke during the period before birth and afterwards. The risk is increased when the mother smokes and when the father smokes. The risk is related to the number of cigarettes smoked, and overall.

Risk increased 2-3 fold or more

Recommendations

We **recommend** that infants should not be exposed to cigarette smoke either before birth or afterwards, and that parents and parents-to-be should be advised of the risk.

Thermal environment and cot death

2.6 In two controlled studies it was shown that infants who died of cot death had been at greater risk of overheating when compared with infants selected as controls. The associated factors were the greater insulation of their clothing and bedding, an increased likelihood of room heating, and a higher ambient temperature.

2.7 There are wide variations in the bedding that mothers put over their infants, even at the same ambient temperature. The normal infant is able to maintain the correct temperature by regulatory mechanisms, an important one being the capability of losing heat from the face and head. There is evidence that a number of factors might impair thermoregulation. They include a high ambient temperature; increased direct heating, for example by the body warmth of others in bed sharing; fever; sleeping on the front; and covering the face and head by wearing a hat or slipping beneath the bedding. It is possible, too, that individual infants are unduly vulnerable to thermal stress at certain periods during their development.

Conclusions

We **conclude** that the risk of cot death is increased when an infant is overwrapped or overheated, especially if feverish or unwell.

> **Risk increased (substantially)**
> (but not yet quantified).

From these observations, together with those on the sleeping position, it is possible to offer guidance on infant care which might lead to a further reduction in the risk of cot death.

Recommendations

We **recommend** that appropriate guidance to parents and others who have responsibility for the care of infants should incorporate the following points:

the room where an infant sleeps should be at a temperature which is comfortable for lightly clothed adults; ie 16-20°C;

indoors, infants need little more bedding than adults;

bedding should not be excessive for the temperature of the room;

bedding should be arranged so that the infant is unlikely to slip underneath, for example, it can be made up so that the infant's feet come down to the end of the cot;

duvets should not be used for an infant under one year;

bedding should not be increased when an infant is unwell or feverish;

an infant should not be exposed to direct heating whilst asleep, for example from a hot water bottle, electric blanket, or radiant heater;

an infant over one month, at home, does not need to be kept as warm as in the hospital baby nursery;

an infant over one month should not wear hats indoors for sleeping unless the room is very cold.

On the other hand, when infants are taken outdoors in cold

weather they can chill rapidly, and it is essential that they are adequately wrapped.

Breast-feeding and cot death

2.8   Breast-feeding has many benefits and few disadvantages, and we strongly **recommend** that breast-feeding be encouraged wherever possible. However, the evidence from published studies does not consistently show that breast-feeding affects the risk of cot death.

Infants who are unwell

2.9   If the sudden unexpected deaths of infants are subjected to thorough investigation, a treatable cause of death is found in a small proportion of them. For these reasons parents, and others who are entrusted with the care of infants, should be encouraged to seek medical advice promptly if an infant is unwell or thought to be unwell. It should, however, be emphasised that the majority of babies who succumb to cot death have not been significantly unwell in the preceding day or two.

Reducing the risk

2.10   It is not claimed that these changes in infant care will eliminate cot death - that will not be possible until the underlying causes and the processes leading to death are better understood - but it will reduce the risks.

2.11   The large majority of babies who are laid on their fronts to sleep do not succumb to cot death, neither are all babies who sleep on their backs spared. The majority of babies who are exposed to cigarette smoke do not die; nor do the great majority of babies who are feverish or unwell. But in every instance - by taking the precautions that we advise - it is possible to reduce the risks.

Monitoring the consequences of interventions

2.12   Studies of specified public interventions in this area of infant care have four kinds of purpose, and all are important in order to guide future action. They are:

(i)　To assess the effectiveness of the national educational campaign ("Back to Sleep") in reaching and being understood by health professionals and the public.

(ii)　To assess changes in infant care practice in respect of sleeping position, exposure to smoking, thermal care, illness management and breast-feeding; and whether they are sustained.

(iii)　To determine whether the changes observed are associated with the predicted changes in the incidence of cot death.

(iv)　To determine whether those changes have significant inadvertent consequences, particularly a shift in the pattern of infant mortality by cause and over time, or significant non-fatal consequences for infants, or for the parents and others who are entrusted with their care.

Recommendations for further action

2.13　We **recommend** that the Department of Health continues to encourage and support programmes to monitor the effectiveness of the "Back to Sleep" campaign, and the consequences; and we commend the action already taken.

2.14　We **recommend** that arrangements be made to detect and assess any changes in mortality during infancy and subsequently attributed to other causes besides cot death, and in significant morbid events including those to parents, in relation to changes in practice; and we welcome the research that has been commissioned.

2.15　We **recommend** that there should be continuing review, to ensure that the benefits of applying the new knowledge to infant care are fully realised, together with monitoring and assessments of the kind described at 2.12.

2.16　We **recommend** that our Report be brought to the notice of the Chief Executive, NHS Management Executive.

Further research

2.17   From the research data available to us it is not to be expected
         that removal of the hazards to which we have drawn attention
         will eliminate cot death. It is likely that there are other factors
         which cannot be influenced without additional knowledge.
         They might include anomalies of physical development that
         confer vulnerabilities upon the infant; physical and biological
         agents (including infectious agents); and social and cultural
         influences whose effects upon infants are poorly understood. It
         will, therefore, be necessary to continue biomedical and health
         service research into cot deaths, and other infant deaths of
         unknown cause.

2.18   We **recommend** that carefully designed and well-conducted
         studies be mounted into the circumstances of unexplained
         infant deaths, the associated socio-biological factors, and the
         pathology of cot death, to learn more of known and possible
         risk factors and their interplay.

2.19   We **recommend** that the attention of the Director of NHS
         Research and Development be drawn to these needs

II. *The Evidence*

1. Sleeping Position and the Risks of Sudden Infant Death Syndrome

Peter J Fleming and Alison J Stewart

Introduction

1.1 The question of whether the infant's sleeping position contributes to the risk of Sudden Infant Death Syndrome (SIDS) has been addressed in many studies over the past 20 years[1]. Although none of the published studies found a lower risk of SIDS for babies sleeping prone, until recently there had been doubts concerning the methodologies of these studies, and there was some resistance within the health care professions to the concept that such a simple practice in infant care, and one which might be so easily amenable to change, could have a major effect.

1.2 The purpose of this paper is to review the published evidence, some of which became available during the preparation of the Report. It forms the background to the recent decision by the United Kingdom Health Departments to recommend that (with particular exceptions) infants should **not** be put to sleep prone.

Published evidence

1.3 The published studies fall into 3 groups:

(i) Retrospective case-control studies
(ii) Prospective studies
(iii) Post-intervention studies

(i) *Retrospective case-control studies*

Over 20 such studies have now been published. The results are summarised in Table 1 and reference[1]. During the 1960s and early 1970s[2,3], the incidence of prone sleeping in the control population was low (<5%) and in studies dating from this time an excess risk was found for infants **not** sleeping supine (ie for infants sleeping prone or on their sides). In all the later

Table 1
Sleeping position of SIDS victims and controls: summary of published controlled studies*

Year	Study No.	No. SIDS	No. Controls	Sleeping Position	Odds Ration (95% C.I.)	p value
(i) Retrospective Studies						
1991	Mitchell[4]	128	503	Prone	5.7 (3.3-10.1)	<0.01
1988	Beal[5]	100	156	Prone	9.3 (4.9-17.6)	<0.01
1986	Cameron[6]	208	393	Prone	3.2 (2.2-4.5)	<0.01
1987	Senecal[7]	20	318	Prone	12.7 (3.6-44.2)	<0.01
1989	Lee[8]	16	32	Prone	11.7 (2.1-66.4)	<0.01
1988	Nicholl[10]	265	273	Prone	2.2 (1.5-3.1)	<0.01
1986	McGlashan[9]	164	329	Prone	1.9 (1.3-2.8)	<0.05
1989	De Jonge[11]	62	254	Prone	4.9 (2.3-10.3)	<0.01
1990	Fleming[12]	67	134	Prone	8.8 (3.4-23.8)	<0.01
1970	Froggatt[2]	148	148	Not Supine	4.2 (2.3-7.8)	<0.01
1972	Carpenter[3]	110	110	Not Supine	2.3 (1.3-4.3)	<0.05
(ii) Prospective Study						
1991	Dwyer[15]	15	116	Prone	4.5 (1.3-15.4)	<0.01
(iii) Post-Intervention Study						
1992	Wigfield[16]	32	64	Prone	9.1 (3.4-24.8)	<0.01

The data have been taken from the publications and used to calculate the odds ratio and p value using Confidence Interval Analysis (BMJ Publications Limited).

published studies the risk of prone sleeping was examined, and compared either with all other sleeping positions or with the risk of sleeping supine.

All of these studies have been criticised[13]. Questions on the position in which a dead infant was found were not, of course, applicable to controls. Moreover, questions on the sleeping position of a dead infant were retrospective and therefore subject to recall bias by parents. Where attempts were made to validate the information on sleeping position given by the parents [12,13], there was no evidence of recall bias. Most importantly a subsequent prospective study[15], with data on sleeping position collected prior to death, showed the same results, as described below.

(ii) *Prospective study*

A single prospective study has been published. The results for a population at high risk of SIDS were very similar to those of the studies described above[15]. Dwyer et al. showed that the prone sleeping position was associated with a risk of SIDS which was 4 times that for other positions when corrected for the confounding effects of other variables (birthweight, maternal age, month of birth).

(iii) *Post-intervention studies*

Two population based post-intervention studies have been reported [16,17,18].

In Holland there was evidence of a rise in SIDS rates during the 1970s and early 1980s, a period during which there was an increase in the proportion of infants sleeping prone. In 1987 a public awareness campaign was launched, aimed at persuading parents not to put their babies down to sleep prone. The proportion of infants sleeping prone fell, from 65% in 1986 to 17% in 1990, and this was accompanied by a fall in the SIDS rate (Fig. 1)[17,18].

In Avon, UK, following a retrospective case-control study which showed that prone sleeping was associated with an 8.8 fold increased risk of SIDS[12], a local public awareness campaign was launched in late 1989. A subsequent study, which included matched controls and a second, random control group of infants prospectively enrolled, showed a fall in the proportion of infants sleeping prone in both of the control groups. There was a parallel fall in the SIDS rate[16]. The initial study showed an association between prone sleeping and SIDS.The subsequent study found that the observed fall in the SIDS rate was very close to that predicted from the initial study for the observed reduction in prone sleeping. This suggests a causal association. The evidence for a causal relationship is strengthened by the results of the second year of the intervention campaign, when a continued fall in the prevalence of prone sleeping was also accompanied by a parallel fall in the SIDS rate (Fig.2).

Related observations

Similar public awareness campaigns in Australia and New Zealand[19] have been followed by falls in SIDS rates, although data on infant sleeping positions before and after these interventions have not yet been published in full. Southall[13] and Gibson[20] pointed out that the SIDS rate has fallen in Scotland in the absence of a concerted publicity campaign. Similar falls have occurred in many English health regions[21], the largest fall occurring in the South West Region. The question of infant sleeping position was the subject of media attention in early 1990 after the publication of the first Avon study[12]. A study from the Isle of Man in 1992[22] showed a pattern of infant sleeping position similar to that observed in Avon. The Isle of Man is isolated from mainland UK and has not been subjected to a planned campaign to change infant care practices. However, media publicity may have influenced the choice of infant sleeping position by parents, and perhaps, most importantly, by midwives, who have a major influence on infant care practices[21]. There is no detailed information on infant sleeping position in the UK prior to this publicity but the striking similarity between the sleeping position of infants in the Isle of Man and in Avon in 1991 suggests that similar changes in patterns of infant sleeping position may have occurred nationally and account, at least in part, for the observed national falls in SIDS rates.

Figure 1.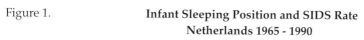

**Infant Sleeping Position and SIDS Rate
Netherlands 1965 - 1990**

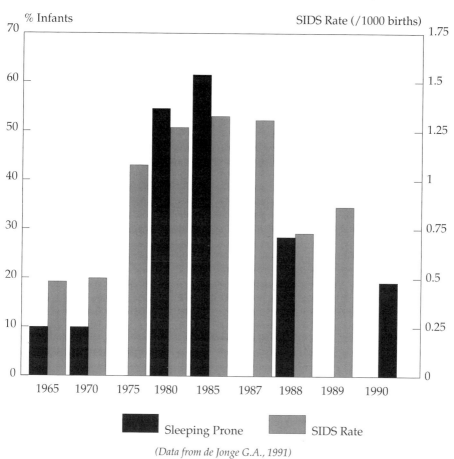

(Data from de Jonge G.A., 1991)

Figure 2.   **Infant Sleeping Position and SIDS Rate**
Avon 1987 - 1992

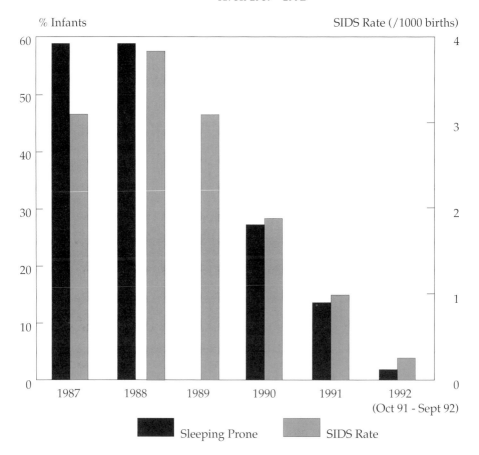

% Infants   SIDS Rate (/1000 births)

Sleeping Prone   SIDS Rate

50

Definition of sleeping position

1.4   In some of the published studies sleeping position was defined as the position in which the infant was put down to sleep; in others it was the position in which the infant was found. Parents only have direct control over the former, so the consideration of avoidable risk will focus on the position in which the infant was put down. This is particularly important for infants put down in the side sleeping position, because it is unstable[16]. Few infants under six months of age who are placed to sleep supine or prone turn over completely in bed. In Avon where mothers are advised to put the lower arm forward when they lay a baby on the side, among infants as young as 6 weeks up to 40% of those who are laid down to sleep on their sides will be found in a different position, the great majority of these having rolled consistently on to their backs, with less than 1% having rolled consistently on to their front[22]. In contrast, 6 (18%) babies found dead in a recent study from Avon had rolled into the prone position from the side position, compared with no control babies. These results give a relative risk of SIDS for side sleeping between 2 and 3 times that of the supine position. From the New Zealand cot death study Mitchell[19] calculated that side sleeping position carried a relative risk of 2.2 (95% CI 1.5-3.1) compared with supine.

1.5   Although there is no firm evidence from prospective studies, there is considerable anecdotal evidence that infants who are placed to sleep in the side position with the lower arm placed well forward of the body are unlikely to roll into the prone position.

1.6   Some of the published studies considered the usual sleeping position of the infant[2,4,6,9,10,15], and others considered the position during the last sleep. This might account for part of the difference in risk attributable to the prone position between these two groups of studies. In general the former studies found a lower relative risk for prone sleeping[1]. Because a greater proportion of infants who usually slept supine were placed prone in their last sleep than vice versa[14], the studies of usual sleeping position would have consistently underestimated the real risk of prone sleeping.

Adverse effects of supine sleeping

1.7   In some countries (eg Czechoslovakia, Hong Kong) the great majority of infants sleep supine, and the SIDS rates are low. Importantly, there is no evidence that choking or aspiration of vomit is a significant problem. In Holland the widespread adoption of the supine sleeping position in 1988 was not followed by any change in the incidence of lethal episodes of aspiration[23]. In Avon during the years 1984-91, during which there were over 750 infant deaths, the only lethal episodes of aspiration outside the newborn period occurred in neurologically impaired infants, all of whom were prone at the time.

1.8   Although there is no evidence that supine sleeping will increase the risk of death from other causes than SIDS in normal infants, there is little evidence on minor adverse effects. It will be important, therefore, to monitor the effects of changes in practice to detect any inadvertent morbid consequences.

1.9   Infants with Pierre-Robin syndrome are at risk of lethal airway obstruction if placed supine, and should always be placed prone for sleep. Newborn infants with respiratory distress, particularly if preterm, commonly have better oxygenation if placed prone[24]. After resolution of the acute respiratory difficulty there is no advantage in continuing the prone position. Infants with gastro-oesophageal reflux vomit more when placed supine than when prone[25], but for most infants this does not seem to impose a significant risk of aspiration. The choice of sleeping position for an infant with clinically significant gastro-oesophageal reflux will depend upon the clinician's assessment of the balance of risks and potential benefits for that individual infant. The suggestion[26] that the head of the cot should be elevated by 10-12 cm to reduce the risk of reflux and hence of aspiration and SIDS, is unsupported by any published data, and may increase the risk of babies slipping under the covers and becoming hot (see 3.9). There has been concern about the risk of the supine sleeping position for infants who are being treated in splints (eg von Rosen splints) for dislocated hips[27], but there is no published evidence that this position is more hazardous to these infants. In the Avon studies there were instances of SIDS in such infants when sleeping prone.

Sleeping position in the newborn period

1.10 SIDS is very uncommon in the first 3 weeks of life and there are few data to assess the relative risks of different sleeping positions at this age. Nonetheless there is some evidence that even at this age the prone position may be associated with increased risk of SIDS[10,17]. But there is no evidence that the risk of aspiration in the supine position is significant for most infants.

1.11 Some newborn infants, particularly if they are preterm, have difficulty in clearing airway secretions and might benefit from the side sleeping position for the first few days of life. Preterm infants with respiratory difficulties might benefit from the prone position. On the other hand, older infants resist attempts to impose a changed sleeping position, and the disadvantage of establishing a practice of prone sleeping might outweigh any conceivable advantage.

Summary

1.12 Over 20 case-control studies from many countries have been published on the association between infant sleeping position and the risk of SIDS. In all of these studies the risk was found to be higher for infants sleeping on the front (prone). Concerns about bias in the original retrospective studies have not been substantiated in a recent prospective study, which confirmed the increased risk associated with sleeping on the front. Reports have now been published from several centres in which attempts were made to change infant sleeping practices. In all of these interventions a reduction in the prevalence of sleeping on the front was accompanied by a fall in the incidence of SIDS. These findings suggest that the relationship is causal.

1.13 In many societies the majority of infants sleep supine (on the back) and there is no evidence of an increased risk of death by aspiration or choking in normal infants.

Conclusions

1.14   We conclude that sleeping on the front is associated with an increased risk of SIDS, the increased risk being 3-8 fold. Why this should be is unclear, but it may be related to airway obstruction or heat stress to which an infant lying on the front may be subject. Evidence on the side sleeping position is limited and inconclusive, but the risk is likely to be between the risks of lying on the front and lying on the back.

1.15   We also conclude that there is no evidence of an increased risk of death by aspiration or choking in normal infants who sleep on the back.

1.16   Some infants (eg those with Pierre-Robin syndrome) should be nursed on the front because of the particular risk of airway obstruction. For others (eg newborn infants with respiratory problems) there might be some temporary advantage from sleeping on the front. In others (eg those with severe gastro-oesophageal reflux) there might be some benefit from sleeping on the front which must be carefully weighed against the increased risk of SIDS. Some newborn infants experience difficulty in clearing airway secretions and might benefit from the side sleeping position for the first few days.

1.17   The practice of placing a rolled up sheet, towel or blanket behind the infant, or of using a wedge to maintain the side position has not been shown to be of value. Such devices might increase the risk of the infant rolling on to the front, although there is now good evidence on the matter.

Recommendations

1.18   We **recommend** that, apart from the exceptions given above (see 1.9-1.11), and once stable respiration has been established, the great majority of infants should be nursed supine (on their backs). If the side position is chosen, the lower arm should be placed well in front of the body to ensure that the infant does not roll prone (on to the front).

1.19   We do **not** recommend placing devices such as wedges and rolled up sheets behind the infant; because doing so might increase the risk of rolling on to the front.

References

1.   Beal SM, Finch CF. An overview retrospective case control studies investigating the relationship between prone sleeping position and SIDS. *J Paediatr Child Health* 1991:27:334-339.

2.   Froggatt P. In: Bergman AR, Beckwith JB, Ray CG (Eds). *Sudden Infant Death Syndrome*. Seattle University of Washington Press. 1970:40.

3.   Carpenter RG. In: Camps FE, Carpenter RG (Eds). *Sudden And Unexpected Deaths In Infancy*. Bristol John Wright. 1972:11.

4.   Mitchell EH, Scragg R, Stewart AW, et al. Results from the first year of the New Zealand cot death study. *NZ Med J* 1991; 104:71-76.

5.   Beal SM. Sleeping position and SIDS. *Lancet* 1988;ii:512.

6.   Cameron MH, Williams AL. Development and testing of scoring systems for predicting infants with high risk of SIDS in Melbourne, Aust. *Paediat J* 1986; suppl 37-45.

7.   Senecal J, Roussey M, Defawe G, et al. Procubitus et mort subite in attendue due nourrisson. *Arch Fr Paediatr* 1987;44:131-136.

8.   Lee N, Chan YF, Davies DP, et al. Sudden Infant Death in Hong Kong: Confirmation of low incidence *BMJ* 1989;298:721.

9.   McGlashan ND. Sleeping position and SIDS. *Lancet* 1986;ii:106

10.   Nicholl JP, O'Cathian A. Sleeping position and SIDS. *Lancet* 1988;ii:106.

11.   DeJonge GA, Engelberts AC, Koomen-Liefting AJM, Kostense PJ. Cot death and prone sleeping in the Netherlands. *BMJ* 1989;298:722.

12.   Fleming PJ, Gilbert R, Azaz Y, et al. Interaction between bedding and sleeping position in the sudden infant death syndrome: a population-based case-control study. *BMJ* 1990;301:85-89.

13.   Southall DP, Samuels MP. Reducing risks in the Sudden Infant Death Syndrome. *BMJ* 1992;304:265-266.

14.   Fleming PJ, Berry PJ, Gilbert R, et al. Interaction between bedding and sleeping position in the sudden death syndrome. *BMJ* 1990;301:494.

15.   Dwyer T, Ponsonby AL, Newman NM, Gibbons LE. Prospective cohort study of prone sleeping and sudden infant death syndrome. *Lancet* 1991;337:1244-1247.

16.   Wigfield RE, Fleming PJ, Berry PJ, et al. Can the fall in Avon's sudden infant death rate be explained by the observed sleeping position changes? *BMJ* 1992;304:282-283.

17.   Engelberts AC. *Cot death in the Netherlands: An epidemiological study.* Thesis ISBN 90-6256-991-9. VU University Press. Amsterdam 1991.

18.   Engelberts AC, De Jonge GA. Choice of sleeping position for infants: possible association with cot death. *Arch Dis Child* 1990;65:462-467.

19.   Mitchell EA, Engelberts AC. Sleeping position and cot deaths. *Lancet* 1991;338:192.

20.   Gibson A, Brooke H, Keeling J. Reduction in sudden infant death syndrome in Scotland. *Lancet* 1991;338:1595.

21.   Gordon RR. Monitoring cot death rates. *BMJ* 1992;304:775-776.

22.   Golding J, Fleming PJ, Parkes S. Cot deaths and sleep position campaigns. *Lancet* 1992;339:748-749.

23.   De Jonge GA. Data supplied from the Netherlands Central Bureau of Statistics on deaths in the Netherlands (ICD E911) of infants under 1 year. 1991.

24.   Martin RJ, Herrell N, Ribin D, Fanaroff A. Effect of supine and prone positions on arterial oxygen tension in the preterm infant. *Paediatrics* 1979;63:528-531.

25.   Orenstein SR, Whittington PT, Orenstein DM. The infant seat as treatment for gastro oesophageal reflux. *N Eng J Med* 1983;309:760-763.

26.   Barrie H. Reducing the risk of cot death. *Arch Dis Child* 1992;67:663.

27.   Report of the SMAC/SNMAC Working Party. Screening for the detection of congenital dislocation of the hip. *Arch Dis Child* 1986;61:921-926.

Parental Smoking and Sudden Infant Death Syndrome

Jean Golding

2.

Introduction

2.1   Epidemiological studies of the sudden infant death syndrome are prone to biases caused by either (a) inadequate identification of cases, and/or (b) inadequate classification of controls. Methodologically more exact are those studies which have started with a large population data base and then identified the children who subsequently died (cohort approach). These studies are usually able to assess the relationship with maternal smoking during pregnancy, but they do not usually have information on paternal smoking or maternal smoking after delivery. For an assessment of these factors therefore a retrospective case-control approach is usually needed. It is useful therefore to compare data collected using each approach.

Published evidence

2.2   The published studies are:

(i)   Prospective cohort studies
(ii) Retrospective case-control studies

(i)   *Prospective Cohort Studies*

A study in Sweden[1] examined all records of postneonatal deaths and identified 190 cases of SIDS. These were compared with 280,000 infants surviving the early neonatal period. Factors from the birth records that were associated with SIDS were taken into account (maternal age, parity, whether the father of the child was living with the mother, sex of the infant, and singleton/multiple birth status) in order to assess the effect of smoking during pregnancy. A strong significant trend was found: compared with mothers who had not smoked during pregnancy, the odds-ratio (OR) for those who had smoked less than 10 cigarettes per day was 1.8 and for those who had smoked 10 or more, the odds-ratio was 2.7. The authors identified a greater effect for infants that had died at less than 68 days (relevant OR 2.8 and 3.6) compared with babies who died at age 68 days or more (OR 1.0 and 2.0)

In the Netherlands[2], the POPS study followed up 1013 infants of either <32 weeks gestation and/or <1500g prospectively. Of these, 15 infants died suddenly and unexpectedly and postmortem showed no obvious cause of death. Of these 15 cases, 80% of mothers had smoked during pregnancy compared with 40% of the rest of the population (OR 6.0, p=0.03). Analysis taking account of maternal age and presence of neonatal hypothermia reduced the odds ratio to 2.39 (p=0.12), but by allowing for hypothermia the analysis might have over-controlled.

In Cardiff, prospectively collected information on the Cardiff birth survey was used to identify factors predictive of SIDS[3]. There was a problem in this study in that the identification of cases was not perfect, and statistical analysis was somewhat inadequate. Nevertheless, the associations found with maternal smoking during pregnancy were striking. Compared with non-smokers, the ORs associated with smoking less than 20 cigarettes per day was 2.2 and for those smoking 20+/day it was 4.8 (p<0.001).

The United States Collaborative Perinatal Project provides important prospective information collected during pregnancy. This study was based on 12 hospitals in different parts of the USA and concerned with births between 1959 and 1966. In all there were 193 cases of SIDS identified using the Beckwith definition[4]. When these were compared with a random sample of 1930 controls selected from the data base, and features such as income, maternal age, parity, the number of antenatal visits, and haematocrit levels taken into account, there was a strong relationship with maternal smoking in pregnancy which gave dose response odds-ratios of: 1.4 (5 cigarettes/day), 1.7 (15 cigarettes/day) and 1.9 (30 cigarettes/day). Nevertheless, there was a strong interaction with maternal anaemia. If the lowest maternal haematocrit level was greater than 30%, there was very little relationship with maternal smoking in pregnancy, but if the maternal haematocrit was less than 30%, the relationship was strong.

A prospective study in California followed 19047 livebirths and identified 44 subsequent cases of SIDS[5]. Smoking during pregnancy was associated with an odds ratio of 4.4, and was the strongest relationship found (p<0.001).

In conclusion, the cohort studies have all shown positive relationships with SIDS, with odds ratios usually at least of the order of 2.0. Wherever the data were available, a dose effect was demonstrated.

(ii) *Retrospective case-control studies*

In Finland[6], a case-control study identified information from maternal records. Deaths had occurred between 1969 and 1980. In all, 52% of 124 SIDS mothers had smoked during pregnancy compared with 21% of 141 controls. Although details are not given in this paper, the information was analysed using log linear regression, and smoking was identified as the most important independent risk factor.

In the UK, a population study in Tameside[7] identified 45 cases of SIDS born between 1982 and 1986 and compared them with 90 next birth controls. Smoking in pregnancy was found to have an odds ratio of 3.32, but adjustments were not made for any social or other factors.

In Avon, Gilbert[8] compared 95 mothers of sudden unexpected deaths with 190 controls. 55% of index mothers reported that they had smoked during pregnancy compared with 33% of controls, giving an odds ratio of 2.5 (p<0.001). For fathers, the relevant figures were 64% of index cases and 39% of controls (OR = 2.78). The numbers of mother smoking after delivery changed only marginally from those smoking during pregnancy. The information was collected by interview of the parents after the death, or of controls when their infants were of a similar age to the SIDS cases. It is possible therefore that there is biased recall in this study. Nevertheless, the ORs are similar to those found in other studies. Dr. Gilbert found that smoking in pregnancy remained an independent risk factor for SIDS after socio-economic status had been taken into account (Gilbert, unpublished MD thesis).

A postal questionnaire to parents of SIDS cases and control infants in the USA related to deaths occurring between 1970 and 1974[9]. The study was confined to white parents and aimed at comparing 100 cases with 100 controls. In the event the response rate was only 56% from cases compared with 86% from controls - the bias in response being wholly associated with parents of cases of SIDS having moved and left no forwarding address. The results of these analyses are therefore very prone to bias. They showed an excess of paternal smoking (53% v 43%) which was not statistically significant; smoking during pregnancy was elicited from 61% of mothers of cases compared with 42% of controls (p<0.05); and 59% of mothers of cases smoked postnatally, compared with 37% of controls (p<0.02). The authors showed that the postnatal smoking effect appeared to be confined to young mothers. Thus for mothers aged under 25, 71% of SIDS compared with 35% of controls were smokers, whereas for mothers over 25, the relative percentages were 41% and 40%. If one looks at the dose response rates in the under 25 year old age group, these gave, for postnatal smoking, an OR of 3.3 for smoking <10 cigarettes/day, 3.9 for 10-19 cigarettes and 7.7 for 20+ cigarettes. A chi-squared for trend gave a p value of less than 0.001. Nevertheless the numbers involved were very small.

In the United States there has been a large case-control multicentre study of SIDS which also showed a strong relationship with smoking in pregnancy[10]. Nevertheless, the case ascertainment was so biased that interpretation of the data was not possible[11].

In Missouri, a study by Malloy[12] of deaths between 1979 and 1983 showed a relative risk of 2.92 for maternal smoking during pregnancy (95% CI, 2.38,3.59).

In Hong Kong SIDS is extremely rare. A case-control study was undertaken however of all cases of SIDS occurring between

1986 and 1987. The 16 cases were compared with 32 controls half of which were hospital matched and half community matched[13]. No cases or controls had mothers who smoked at all (indeed it is culturally unacceptable for mothers to smoke in Hong Kong), but 50% of fathers of cases smoked compared with 22% of the controls (OR=3.5).

In Tasmania a study between 1980 and 1986 compared 167 SIDS cases with 334 next birth controls, matched for hospital and sex[14]. The odds ratios found were -for paternal smoking 1.73 (p=0.05, for 'usual' maternal smoking 2.98 (p<0.001), for smoking during pregnancy 3.32 (p<0.001), and postnatal smoking 2.20 (p<0.01). The numbers were unfortunately too small to look at dose response levels.

A large New Zealand study which is currently under way is identifying cases of SIDS in the whole national population[15]. From their first report of 162 cases of SIDS compared with 589 controls, the odds ratio for smoking during pregnancy was 2.73 (p<0.001), whereas for postnatal smoking the odds ratio was 2.91. For postnatal smoking the authors broke down the dose response relationship and found that in comparison with non-smokers, the odds ratio was 1.87 for mothers smoking 1-9 cigarettes/day, 2.64 for those smoking 10-19 and 5.06 for those smoking 20+ cigarettes. A large multivariate analysis then took account of maternal education, number of antenatal visits, marital status, admission to special care baby unit, parity, social class, birthweight, gestation, race and maternal age and showed the odds ratio for postnatal smoking as 1.85. In addition to these factors they then took account of breast feeding and sleeping position and showed the postnatal smoking odds ratio had fallen to 1.83. From their data they calculated the population attributable risk to be 40%. They give no reason for concentrating on postnatal smoking as opposed to antenatal smoking in this study.

Perhaps the most important information, however, is derived from the Sheffield multicentre study[16]. The authors looked first at the unadjusted odds ratios of the smoking habits of the mother during pregnancy and her partner postnatally.

Table 2.1 **Smoking habits of parents and risk of cot death**

Mother (during pregnancy)	Partner (after the birth)	Odds Ratio
Non-smoker	Non-smoker	1.0 reference value
Non-smoker	**Smoker**	1.39
Smoker	Non-smoker	1.68
Smoker	**Smoker**	3.46

Logistic regression identified independent effects for maternal smoking (OR = 2.13) and paternal smoking (OR = 1.63). Like other authors they showed that the maternal smoking effect was most strongly related to the early SIDS deaths (<8 weeks). Paternal smoking, in contrast, appeared to be associated with the later deaths.

These effects were statistically highly significant, they remained after controlling for maternal age, gravidity, housing repair and birthweight.

Summary

2.3   There have been five cohort studies in which information on maternal smoking was collected prospectively. All showed a strong, consistent and statistically significant relationship between maternal smoking and the risk of SIDS. Moreover, the risk was dose dependent. Similar results have been obtained from case-control studies in which information was collected retrospectively. There is also evidence from three studies that passive smoking may be important. The separate contributions to the risk of SIDS of maternal smoking in pregnancy, passive smoking in pregnancy, and passive smoking postnatally have not yet been determined.

Conclusions

2.4   From a review of the literature there is substantial evidence that sudden infant death syndrome is strongly associated with a history of maternal smoking. There are clear dose response effects.

2.5 Because most women who smoke during pregnancy also smoke postnatally it is impossible at this stage to say whether the effect is prenatal or postnatal. Nevertheless, associations with paternal smoking in three studies [13,14,16] indicate that there may be a passive smoking effect as well. The latter could operate either prenatally or postnatally.

2.6 The effects of maternal smoking may well be a biologically plausible cause of SIDS. A study on 295 infants in Oklahoma showed an increased rate of central apnoea in infants whose mothers had smoked during pregnancy ($p<0.01$), and that this relationship was still apparent after allowance had been made for gestation, birthweight, maternal age, and caffeine consumption. The relationship with postnatal maternal smoking was non-significant ($p=0.06$)[17].

2.7 The crucial question is whether the associations demonstrated here are causal. Bradford Hill[18] has identified a number of criteria which make causality likely. These include the strength of associations, their consistency, biological plausibility and a dose-response relationship. All have been demonstrated for maternal smoking and SIDS. It therefore seems very likely that there is a causal relationship between maternal smoking and SIDS. Whether the relationship is with antenatal or postnatal smoking is not clear.

Recommendations

2.8 We **recommend** that babies should not be exposed to cigarette smoke either before birth or afterwards, and that parents and parents-to-be should be advised.

References

1.   Haglund B, Cnattingius S. Cigarette smoking as a risk factor for sudden infant death syndrome: a population-based study. *American Journal of Public Health* 1990; 80: 29-32.

2.   Wierenga H, Brand R, Geudeke T, et al. Prenatal risk factors for cot death in very preterm and small-for-gestational-age infants. *Early Human Development* 1990; 23: 15-26.

3.   Murphy FJ, Newcombe RG, Sibert JR. The epidemiology of sudden infant death syndrome. *J Epidem Comm Health* 1982; 36: 17-21.

4.   Bulterys MG, Greenland S, Kraus JF. Chronic fetal hypoxia and sudden infant death syndrome: interaction between maternal smoking and low hematocrit during pregnancy. *Pediatrics* 1990; 86: 535-540.

5.   Lewak N, van den Berg BJ, Beckwith JB. Sudden infant death syndrome risk factors. *Clinical Pediatrics* 1979; 18: 405-11.

6.   Rintahaka PJ, Hirvonen J. The epidemiology of sudden infant death syndrome in Finland 1969-1980. *Forensic Science International* 1986; 30: 219-233.

7.   McLoughlin A. Sudden infant deaths in Tameside. *Health Visitor* 1988; 61: 235-237.

8.   Gilbert R. Unpublished MD thesis.

9.   Bergman AB, Wiesner LA. Relationship of passive cigarette-smoking to sudden infant death syndrome. *Pediatrics* 1976: 58:665-668.

10.   Hoffman HJ, Hunter JC, Ellish NJ et al. *Adverse reproductive factors and the sudden infant death syndrome.*In: Harper RM, Hoffman HJ, (eds) Sudden Infant Death Syndrome. Risk Factors and Basic Mechanisms. New York: PMA Publishing Corp, 1988: 153-175.

11.   Unsigned editorial. Choice of cases - with special reference to SIDS. *Paediatric & Perinatal Epidemiology* 1991; 5: 1-3.

12. Malloy MH, Kleinman JC, Land GH et al. The association of maternal smoking with age and cause of infant death. *American Journal of Epidemiology* 1988; 128: 46-55.

13. Lee NNY, Chan YF, Davies DP, et al. Sudden infant death syndrome in Hong Kong: confirmation of low incidence. *BMJ* 1989; 298; 721-722.

14. McGlashan MD. Sudden infant deaths in Tasmania, 1980-1986: A 7 year prospective study. *Social Science & Medicine* 1989; 29: 1015-1026.

15. Mitchell EA, Scragg R, Stewart AW, et al. Cot death supplement. Results from the first year of the New Zealand Cot Death Study. *NZ Med J* 1991; 104: 71-76.

16. Nicholl JP, O'Cathain A. *Antenatal smoking, postnatal passive smoking, and sudden infant death syndrome.* In: Effects of Smoking on the Fetus, Neonate and Child. Ed Poswillo D, Alberman E. Oxford: Oxford Medical Publications 1992.

17. Toubas PL, Duke JC, McCaffree MA, et al. Effects of maternal smoking and caffeine habits of infantile apnoea: a restrospective study. *Pediatrics* 1986; 78: 159-163.

18. Hill A Bradford. Principles of Medical Statistics 8th Edn. London: *Lancet* 1966.

Thermal Environment and Sudden Infant Death Syndrome

Christopher J Bacon

Introduction

3.1   Sustained exposure to temperatures outside the range of tolerance of the human body can cause death at any age. Deaths in infancy have been recorded following exposure to cold in unheated rooms on winter nights[1] and also following exposure to high temperatures generated in cars parked in the sun[2,3]. Such deaths can appropriately be ascribed to hypothermia and to heatstroke respectively, and do not come into the category of Sudden Infant Death Syndrome (SIDS). However, it has been suggested that thermal environments that are less obviously extreme may also cause or contribute to sudden death in infancy. In these cases, where the causal link would not be clear, death might be attributed to SIDS.

Hypothermia and SIDS

3.2   The well-known association of SIDS with cold weather[4] might suggest that hypothermia was the operative factor. However, there are not published studies showing that a lower ambient temperature or less insulation are risk factors for SIDS. Furthermore, there is evidence that the thermal environment of sleeping infants tends, paradoxically, to be warmer in winter than in summer because of the use of room heating and thicker insulation[5,6].

Hyperthermia and SIDS

3.3   For some years there have been suggestions that overheating, whether because of a high ambient temperature or excessive insulation, or both, may be a cause of SIDS, but until recently the evidence has been mainly circumstantial or anecdotal.

Published evidence

3.4   Two controlled studies have now been published, the first from Avon[7] the second from Tasmania[8].

(i) *Case-control studies*

The Avon study examined insulation and room heating in 64 cases of SIDS and 128 matched controls. The average insulation of the bedding and clothing of the SIDS cases was 1.1 tog more than that for controls (95% confidence interval 0.15 -2.2, p = 0.025), and the relative risk for SIDS was 1.14 per tog above 8 togs (95% confidence interval 1.02 to 1.28, p < 0.05). There was a marked difference between 24 SIDS victims aged <70 days and 38 aged >70 days. In the younger group there was no significant difference in insulation between index cases and controls, whereas in the older group the mean difference was 2.39 tog (p < 0.01). With regard to room heating, the heating had been left on all night in the homes of a significantly higher proportion of SIDS infants than of controls (28/67 vs 34/134: relative risk 2.7, 95% confidence interval 1.4 to 5.2, p < 0.01). It has been shown that, for a given outside temperature, bedrooms that are heated all night are on average 4°C warmer than unheated bedrooms[5].

The Tasmanian study, which compared 28 cases of SIDS with 54 matched controls, used different methodology but showed similar results. Mean insulation for SIDS cases was 1.3 tog more than for controls (p = 0.05), and the relative risk for a 1 tog increase in insulation was 1.17 (95% confidence interval 0.99 to 1.38). The ambient temperature for SIDS cases was measured by the attendant ambulance crew (by which time the temperature might have altered from that at the time of death). The mean value was 18.1°C for SIDS cases and 16.6°C for controls (p = 0.15), and the relative risk for a 5°C increase in ambient temperature was 1.57 (95% confidence interval 0.85 to 2.91). SIDS cases were also more likely to have had room heating than matched controls (relative risk 10.5, 95% confidence interval 1.3 to 85.05). Insulation was related to ambient temperature by expressing measured insulation in terms of its difference from the theoretical ideal insulation for the measured ambient temperature. The mean ± SD value for excess insulation thus calculated was significantly greater for SIDS cases than for controls (2.3 ± 3.4 vs 0.6 ± 2.3 tog; $p = 0.009$). However, the calculation is open to criticism because the formula used to determine ideal insulation has not been validated in infants.

(ii) Intervention study

In the only intervention study reported to date, Stanton[9] noted a fall in the incidence of SIDS in Scarborough Health District from 23 cases in the 3 years (1983-1985) preceding to 13 cases in the 4 years (1987-1990) following a campaign of advice to parents about room temperature and insulation. This difference was highly significant ($p = 0.0023$), but the numbers were small and it was not possible to be certain that the reduction in SIDS resulted specifically from the intervention, especially when from 1989 onward there was a falling incidence nationally.

Effect of insulation alone

3.5   Although the two case-control studies both found that high insulation was a risk factor for SIDS, the risk demonstrated was small, and there is evidence that infants in normal circumstances are able to tolerate a very wide range of insulation. A population study of 649 infants in Newcastle showed that mothers varied greatly in the bedding they put on them at the same ambient temperature[5]. At a room temperature of 17°C, for example, infants were given insulation ranging from 3.2 to 42 tog, and none seemed any the worse for it. Anderson and colleagues showed that infants who were heavily insulated were able to maintain a normal temperature by losing more heat from their heads[10], and Kerslake has demonstrated that increases in bedding above a certain level do not give a proportionate increase in effective insulation[11]. It therefore seems unlikely that high insulation *per se* is a cause of SIDS.

Other factors in thermal balance

3.6   Other determinants of thermal balance, such as ambient temperature, fever as a result of infection, sleeping position, direct heating to the infant, and covering of the head, may each have an important effect that interacts with that of insulation.

3.7   Many studies have shown that often SIDS victims have had a minor infection. In Avon insulation and infection were studied in 68 victims of sudden unexpected death (most of whom were categorised as SIDS) and compared with 136 matched controls[12]. The 10 SIDS babies with viral infections had significantly higher mean insulation than the 8 controls with similar infections (11.0 vs 5.6 tog; p = 0.0016), whereas there was no significant difference between the insulation of SIDS victims and controls without viral infection. Similar differences in insulation were found between the index cases and controls with bacterial infection. The combination of high insulation and infection gave a much greater risk of SIDS than either alone. If substantiated in further studies this suggests that the link between infection and SIDS may sometimes lie in disturbed thermal balance. The likelihood of such an interaction will be increased by the tendency of mothers to put on more bedding when the infant has an infection[5].

3.8   Sleeping on the front (prone) is now accepted as a risk factor for SIDS. The reason for this increased risk is not yet established, but one suggestion is that the prone position may increase the tendency for an infant to become overheated[13]. This idea is supported by the finding in the Avon study[7] of a greater risk for SIDS among infants sleeping prone if they were heavily insulated. The Avon study found that the relative risk for prone infants with insulation >10 tog was much greater than for those with insulation <6 tog.

3.9   There appear to have been no studies of the effect on an infant's thermal balance of direct heating, the commonest form of which is the warmth from another body (or bodies) during bed-sharing. Several reports allude to SIDS while bed-sharing[12] but none has examined the question in depth. A recent study in Newcastle (unpublished) found that 7 out of 41 (17%) SIDS victims were in their parents' bed when they died, in contrast to 15 out of 649 (2.3%) infants surveyed in the general population (p <0.001). The link between bed-sharing and SIDS is highly complex, and the possible contribution of hyperthermia must await further study.

3.10   Total covering of an infant's head may have a critical effect on thermal balance, because it has been demonstrated that the uncovered head provides the main channel for losing extra heat when a baby is heavily insulated[10]. Total covering of the head most commonly occurs when an infant slips down underneath the bedding. Although there are no reports that specifically examine this factor, the Newcastle study found that 9 out of 41 (22%) SIDS victims had become totally covered in this way, as compared with 5 out of 649 (0.8%) babies of the same age in the general population (p <0.001). Similarly, in the Avon study, 23 out of 95 victims of sudden unexpected death were found with their heads covered, either by the bedding or by a hat[12], in contrast with none in the control group. It is also possible that part of the risk of the prone position may reside in the greater tendency for prone babies to slip down under their bedding. Although there is not firm evidence on this point there is an impression that babies are more likely to slip down under duvets than blankets.

Possible mechanism

3.11   The mechanism by which overheating might lead to SIDS is undetermined. Apnoea seems the most likely possibility[15,16].

3.12   The characteristic age range for SIDS could be explained, in the over-heating hypothesis, by the lower metabolic rate of infants in the early weeks of life[17], and by the increasing ability to make effective protective responses after 3 months of age. Alternatively, the critical response to overheating could be age-specific, as is the case for febrile convulsions. There might also be variations in the individual response and a thermal stress that was innocuous for one infant could be dangerous for another.

Sweating

3.13   SIDS victims are sometimes found soaked in sweat, suggesting that they were trying to lose surplus heat before they died. It is reasonable to suppose that visible sweating is a useful indicator that an infant is too hot. However the accuracy of this sign has not been established: it might vary, for example, with individual response and with ambient humidity.

Summary

3.14   In two controlled studies infants who died of SIDS were shown
        to have been at greater risk of overheating when compared with
        infants selected as controls. The associated factors were the
        greater insulation provided by their clothing and bedding, more
        likelihood of room heating, and a higher ambient temperature

Conclusions

3.15   The two published controlled studies point to a small added
        risk for SIDS from high insulation and from high ambient
        temperature. No studies show the contrary. There is also much
        anecdotal evidence suggesting a link between overheating and
        SIDS. High insulation *per se* is unlikely to cause SIDS but might
        do so through an interaction with other factors that contribute
        to an infant's thermal balance; in particular ambient
        temperature, fever, sleeping position, direct heating and
        covering of the head. The only published intervention study is
        not conclusive, and a definitive study may now be impossible
        because of the various national interventions already begun.

3.16   From the evidence available it is possible to give balanced
        advice to parents about those aspects of infants' thermal
        environment that are most amenable to control. Besides the
        possibility that some deaths might thereby be prevented,
        mothers are clearly in need of guidance on this aspect of infant
        care[5].

Recommendations

3.17   We **recommend** that infants should not be overwrapped or
        overheated, especially when they are feverish or unwell.

3.18   We **recommend** that guidance to parents and others who have
        responsibilities for the care of infants incorporates the following
        points:

the room where an infant sleeps should be at a temperature which is comfortable for lightly clothed adults, ie16-20°C;

indoors, infants need little more bedding than adults;

bedding should not be excessive for the temperature of the room;

bedding should be arranged so that the infant is unlikely to slip underneath; for example, it can be made up so that the infant's feet come down to the end of the cot;

duvets should not be used for infants under one year;

bedding should not be increased when the infant is unwell or feverish;

whilst asleep an infant should not be exposed to direct heating; for example, from a hot water bottle, electric blanket, or radiant heater;

an infant over one month, at home, does not need to be kept as warm as in the hospital nursery;

an infant over one month should not wear hats indoors for sleeping unless the room is very cold.

3.19   On the other hand, when infants are taken outdoors in cold weather they can chill rapidly, and it is essential that they be adequately wrapped.

References

1.   Arneil G C, Kerr M M. Severe hypothermia in Glasgow infants in winter. *Lancet* 1963; i:758-9.

2.   Wadlington W B, Tucker V L., Fly F, Freen HS. Heatstroke in infancy. *Am. J Dis Child* 1976; 130: 1250-1251.

3.   King K, Negus K, Vance J C. Heat stress in motor vehicles: a poblem in infancy. *Paediatrics* 1981; 68: 579-582.

4.   Murphy M F G, Campbell M J. Sudden infant death syndrome and environmental emperature: an analysis using vital statistics. *J Epidemiol Community Health* 1987; 41: 63-71.

5.   Bacon C J, Bell S A, Clulow E E et al. How mothers keep their babies warm. *Arch Dis Child* 1991; 66: 627-632.

6.   Fleming P, Azaz Y, Wigfield R et al. *Laboratory and community studies of thermal balance in infants: possible relevance to SIDS.* Proc. 2nd SIDS Internat Conf. Ed Walker A. Perinatology Press, New York 1992 (in press).

7.   Fleming P J, Gilbert R, Azaz Y et al. Interaction between bedding and sleeping position in the sudden infant death syndrome: a population based case-control study. *BMJ* 1990; 301: 85-89.

8.   Ponsonby A-L, Dwyer T, Gibbons L E et al. Thermal environment and sudden infant death syndrome: case-control study. *BMJ* 1992; 304: 277-282.

9.   Stanton A N. Avoiding overheating and preventing cot death (letter). *Lancet* 1991; ii: 1144.

10.   Anderson E S, Wailoo M P, Petersen S A. Use of thermographic imaging to study babies sleeping at home. *Arch Dis Child* 1990; 1266-67.

11.   Kerslake D McK. The insulation provided by infants' bedclothes. *Ergonomics* 1991; 34: 893-907.

12.   Gilbert R E, Rudd P T, Berry P J et al. Combined effect of infection and heavy wrapping in sudden infant death. *Arch Dis*

Child 1992; 67: 171-177.

13. Nelson E A S, Taylor B J, Weatherall I L. Sleeping position and infant bedding may predispose to hyperthermia and the sudden infant death syndrome. *Lancet* 1989; i: 199-201.

14. Luke J L. Sleeping arrangements of Sudden Infant Death Syndrome victims in the District of Columbia - a preliminary report. *Jnl For Sci* 1978; 23 (2): 379-383.

15. Gozal D, Colin A A, Daskalovic Y I, Jaffe M. Environmental overheating as a cause of transient respiratory chemoreceptor dysfunction in an infant. *Pediatrics* 1988; 82: 738-740.

16. Levine M R, Fleming P J, Azaz Y, McCabe R. Changes in breathing pattern accompanying environmental cooling in human infants [Abstract]. *Early Hum Dev* 1989; 19: 216-217.

17. Azaz Y, Fleming P J, Levine M R, et al. *The relationship between environmental temperature, metabolic rate sleep state and evaporative water loss in infants from birth to three months.* Ped Research 1992 (in press).

4. Breast-feeding and Sudden Infant Death Syndrome

Jean Golding

Introduction

4.1   Various studies have looked at the relationship between breast-feeding and Sudden Infant Death Syndrome (SIDS). As with smoking more weight should be given to population-based prospective cohort studies than to retrospective case-control studies. Most important, too, are other factors taken into account in the analyses. For the most part these have been inadequate. For example, mothers who smoke during pregnancy are less likely to intend breast-feeding, and those who start breast-feeding are less likely to succeed than non-smoking mothers[12]. Babies born preterm are at increased risk of SIDS yet are less likely to be breast-fed. Therefore it is not surprising that studies which have not taken these factors into account appear to show a protective effect with breast-feeding.

Published evidence

4.2   The study design that is least prone to bias records information gathered during the child's life rather than after death has taken place. This is a prospective cohort study. Two such studies have looked at SIDS. They are American National Collaborative Perinatal Project and the Oxford Record Linkage Study. Many more studies have used the case-control approach, obtaining information on breast-feeding by asking the mother after her child is born. Although less costly these studies are prone to bias, and consequently less accurate.

(i) Prospective studies

The American National Collaborative Perinatal Project followed up 50,000 children from birth. Those who died and whose deaths were attributed to SIDS were compared with the remaining children. There was a lower incidence of breast-feeding among cases of SIDS. The authors suggested that this could be largely explained by maternal education and prematurity, both SIDS and bottle-feeding being more prevalent among families with low levels of education and premature infants. They did not adjust for smoking[1].

The Oxford Record Linkage study identified all cases of SIDS occurring in a large population of births. In two studies, which related respectively to births in the periods 1966-1970 and 1971-1975, after matching for maternal age, parity, social class and marital status there was no difference in the onset of breast-feeding between cases and controls[2,3].

(ii) Case-control studies

The large American study, the NICHD SIDS cooperative epidemiological study, included large numbers of cases and controls but had a subjective bias in its case ascertainment[4]. It was possible that cases that were of lower social status would be preferentially included in this study. Such a bias did not occur with the controls and therefore the results are questionable. Certainly this study found that the proportion of SIDS cases that had been breast-fed at all was lower than among controls. For blacks the figures were 17% as opposed to 27% controls, and for whites 35% as opposed to 58%. These differences were statistically significant and stayed significant once account had been taken of maternal age, parity and social class. Nevertheless the inherent biases in this study make interpretation impossible[5].

In a study in New Zealand of SIDS cases in 1987-1988, 83% had been breast-fed ever, compared with 92% of controls. At discharge from obstetric hospital 66% of index cases against 85% of controls were solely breast-fed. This was highly significant after allowing for ante-natal classes, ante-natal care, maternal education, marital status, admission to special care, parity, social class, birthweight, gestation, race, season, maternal age, smoking and sleeping postion[6].

This result contrasts with the results of recent studies from Avon where no significant difference was shown between breast-feeding by the mothers of infants dying of SIDS compared with controls[7].

Earlier information from Britain had confirmed that SIDS cases were less likely to be breast-fed on discharge from hospital than controls. In a study from nine areas of Southern England, 53% of SIDS cases were breast-fed on discharge compared with 68% of controls but no account had been taken of social or other factors to see whether they explained the difference. The authors found that in those homes classified as excellent, there was less breast-feeding in the cases than in the controls, but in poorer homes, the proportion of cases and controls breast-fed was equivalent. Once again these data are difficult to interpret[8].

An early study based in London and Cambridge between 1958-1961 found that 74% of 110 cases compared with 84% of 196 controls were breast-feeding soon after delivery. Again there was no attempt to take other factors into account and interpretation is difficult[9].

In Hong Kong, an area with an exceptionally low incidence of SIDS, breast-feeding is very rare. Indeed, of the 16 SIDS cases there were none that had been breast-fed at all, and on 32 controls only 2 had been breast-fed[10].

A most rigorous study in regard to ascertainment of feeding history was conducted in Copenhagen. 131 cases of SIDS which occurred between 1956-1971 were compared with 4 times the number of controls whose histories had been taken from Health Visitor records. Social factors were not taken into account. By the 2nd week of life 80% of SIDS cases and 92% of controls were being breast-fed; by one month the figures were 53% and 79%; and by 2 months they were 23% and 55%. Over time there had been a fall in the incidence of breast-feeding, but no change in the rate of SIDS. Because none of the mechanisms suggested for explaining a negative association with breast-feeding seemed to fit the facts, the association with breast-feeding was thought to be an artifact. One of the most cogent findings that persuaded the authors that there was no association with breast feeding was that the age distribution at death of children who had been breast-fed was exactly the same as that of the deaths of those who had not. They also suggested that if death was related to an overwhelming infection, against which infants who had more prolonged breast-feeding would have correspondingly longer protection then such SIDS cases who had been breast-fed would have lived longer. The authors concluded that differences in breast-feeding between SIDS cases and controls merely reflected other features that were associated with SIDS[11].

Summary

4.3   Unlike the information available on sleeping position and on smoking in pregnancy, the information in regard to breast-feeding and SIDS is inconsistent. Whilst breast-feeding has many important beneficial effects, it is not evident that SIDS is prevented by breast feeding.

4.4   One of the major factors that influences breast-feeding rates appears to be maternal smoking habit. Mothers who smoke are not only less likely to start breast-feeding, but having started they are more likely to stop early. Very few of the studies of breast-feeding and SIDS have taken account of smoking at all. Without smoking being taken into account however positive associations of SIDS with artificial feeding must remain questionable. There remain the data from New Zealand which appear to show a marked increase in risk in babies who have not been breast-fed. The breast-feeding rate as a whole is high in New Zealand, and mothers who do not breast-feed are exceptional in a number of ways. It may well be that these are the important features in relation to SIDS rather than breast-feeding itself.

Conclusions

4.5   Breast-feeding has many benefits and few disadvantages. However, it is not clear from published studies that breast-feeding affects the risk of SIDS.

Recommendations

4.6   We strongly **recommend** that breast-feeding be encouraged wherever possible.

References

1. Kraus JF, Greenland S, Bulterys M. Risk factors for sudden infant death syndrome in the US collaborative perinatal project. *Inter. Journal of Epidemiology* 1989; 18: 113-120.

2. Fredrick J. Sudden unexpected death in the Oxford record linkage area. Details of pregnancy, delivery and abnormality in the infant. *Brit J Prev Soc Med* 1974; 28: 164-71.

3. Golding J, Limerick S, Macfarlane A. *Sudden Infant Death Patterns, puzzles and problems*. Somerset, England: Open Books Publishing Limited, 1985.

4. Damus K, Pakter J, Krongrad E, et al. *Postnatal medical and epidemiological risk factors or the sudden infant death syndrome. In: 'Sudden Infant Death Syndrome, risk factors and basic mechanisms'.* Eds. Harper, RM, Hoffman, HJ 1988: 187-201.

5. Editorial. Choice of cases - with special reference to SIDS. *Paediatric & Perinatal Epid* 1991; 5:1-3.

6. Mitchell EA, Scragg R, Stewart AW, Becroft DMO, et al. Cot death supplement. Results from the first year of the New Zealand cot death study. *NZ Med J* 1991; 104: 71-76.

7. Gilbert R. Unpublished MD Thesis.

8. Watson E, Gardner A, Carpenter RG. An epidemiological and sociological study of unexpected death in infancy in nine areas of Southern England. *Med, Sci, Law,* 1981; 21: 78-88.

9. Carpenter RG, Shaddick CW. Role of infection, suffociation, and bottle feeding in cot death. *Brit J Prev Soc Med* 1965; 19: 1-7.

10. Davies DP, Chan YF, Lau E, et al. Sudden infant death syndrome in Hong Kong: confirmation of low incidence. *BMJ* 1989; 298: 721.

11. Biering-Sorensen F, Jorgensen T, Hidden J. Sudden infant death in Copenhagen 1956-1971: 1 Infant feeding. *Acta Paed Scand* 1978; 67: 129-137.

12.   Office of Population Censuses and Surveys. *Infant feeding* 1990. London: HMSO, 1992.

The Chief Medical Officer's Expert Group on the Sleeping Position of Infants and Cot Death

Dr Eileen D Rubery PhD FRCR MRCPath (Chairman)
Department of Health, London.

Dr Christopher J Bacon FRCP
Consultant Paediatrician, Friarage Hospital, Northallerton, North Yorkshire.

Mrs A Barnes RGN
Nurse Manager, Ealing Hospital, London.

Ms Mary Broadhurst RGN RM
Director of Midwifery Services, Bexley Health Authority, Kent.

Dr Shireen Chantler PhD
Secretary, Scientific Advisory Committee, Foundation for the Study of Infant Deaths, London.

Dr Brian R B Cooke MFPHM
Health Education Authority, London.

Dr Peter J Fleming FRCP FRCP(C)
Consultant Paediatrician, Royal Hospital for Sick Children, Bristol.

Mrs Elizabeth Fradd RGN
Director of Children's Nursing, Nottingham Health Authority, Nottingham.

Professor Jean Golding PhD FSS
Professor of Paediatric and Perinatal Epidemiology, Department of Child Health, Royal Hospital for Sick Children, Bristol.

Dr Edmund N Hey DPhil DM FRCP
Consultant Paediatrician, Princess Mary Maternity Hospital, Newcastle upon Tyne.

Professor Richard J Madeley DM FFCM
Department of Community Medicine and Epidemiology, University of Nottingham Medical School, Nottingham.

Ms Alison Stewart RGN
Royal Hospital for Sick Children, Bristol.

Observers

Dr Bernadette Fuge MB
Welsh Office.

Mrs Felicity Leenders BA RGN RM RHV
Department of Health, London.

Dr Margaret A R Thomson MRCOG
Scottish Home and Health Department.
(Until May 1992).

Dr Brian T A Potter MRCGP
Scottish Home and Health Department.
(From May 1992).

Dr Heather J Kilgore MB DObst RCOG
Department of Health and Social Services, Northern Ireland.
(Until May 1992).

Dr Adrian P Mairs FRCS
Department of Health and Social Services, Northern Ireland.
(From May 1992).

Dr Elizabeth J Wilson MRCP FRCR
Research Management Divisision, Department of Health,
London.
(Until May 1992).

Dr Rudolph B. Singh MB MSc
Research Management Division, Department of Health,
London.
(From May 1992)

Secretariat

Dr Ian A F Lister Cheese PhD FRCP
Department of Health, London.

Mr John Crook
Department of Health, London.

Miss Joanne Shipton
Department of Health, London.

Professional Advice from the Chief Medical Officers and Chief Nursing Officers of United Kingdom Health Departments.

Professional letters (Sleeping Position of Infants and the Risk of Cot Death (Sudden Infant Death)) were issued by the Chief Medical Officer (CMO) and Chief Nursing Officer (CNO) of each of the United Kingdom Health Departments. The text of the letter from the Department of Health (PO/CMO(91) 16,PL/CNO(91)11) is given. Similar letters were issued by the CMOs and CNOs of Wales, Scotland and Northern Ireland.

November 1991

Dear Doctor/Nursing Officer,

Sleeping Position of Infants and the Risk of Cot Death (Sudden Infant Death)

Each year there are 1200-1400 cot deaths in England (about 2 per 1000 liveborn infants). These deaths are sudden, unexpected and they are unexplained. Although the incidence and circumstances of cot deaths vary between countries, and change over time, a number of factors have been shown to be associated with an increased risk of cot death. But in many instances such factors are absent.

The purpose of this letter is to draw your attention to recommendations received from a group of experts who were asked to consider the evidence relating to the sleeping position of infants and the risk of cot death. The group have concluded that the risk of cot death can be reduced if babies are not placed prone (on their front) when they are laid down to sleep.

The group also concluded that there was no evidence that placing healthy babies on their back results in an increased risk of death from choking or vomiting.

In particular circumstances babies may need to be nursed prone. These include some babies in hospital in special care, babies with severe gastro-oesophageal reflux, babies receiving treatment in splints for unstable hips, and babies with Pierre Robin syndrome. It will be important for doctors and nurses to

86

explain why the prone position is best for these babies.

These conclusions were passed to the public forthwith, by a press statement, a copy of which accompanies this letter.

Background

Recent research suggests that babies who are laid prone to sleep are at greater risk of cot death than those laid on the side or supine. Importantly, in reports from the Netherlands and preliminary reports of studies from New Zealand, Australia and this country, not yet published, a reduction in the use of the prone position has been accompanied by a fall in the incidence of cot death. Babies who are laid on the side are more likely to roll over on to the front, and the supine position may therefore be preferable. Alternatively the underneath arm may be placed forward to prevent the baby rolling into the prone position.

The cause of the risk attributable to the prone position is not understood but may relate to several factors. They include upper airways obstruction should a baby turn the head face down; and the important role of the face in thermal control in babies, especially if they are overwrapped or in a very hot room, and particularly if the metabolic rate is increased by infection.

As babies grow older they start to take up the position that is most comfortable to them. From 4 to 5 months many babies turn themselves over when they are awake. From 6 to 7 months many babies turn over while they are asleep and may adopt a position which is no different from that in which they are placed to sleep. There is no need for concern about a baby taking up a prone position in these circumstances. The incidence of cot death falls rapidly after 5-6 months.

Some babies who are accustomed to sleeping prone will not tolerate a change in sleeping position and may be difficult to settle if placed on the side or supine - in such cases it is probably wise not to distress the baby by insisting on the new position.

There has been much speculation about the causes of cot death, often without a sound scientific basis. This has been confusing for parents who have not always known what was best for their baby. It has also caused distress to bereaved parents. It is not possible to avoid all cot deaths while the underlying causes remain unexplained, but it is possible to reduce the risk. *Sleeping position is only one factor*. Others include the risks associated with cigarette smoke and the risks of overheating a baby.

Finally it is common sense to encourage everyone to seek professional advice speedily if a baby seems unwell.

The Health Education Authority has taken immediate action. It is arranging for the texts of the Pregnancy Book (page 72) and Birth to Five (page 19) to be brought into line with the new advice. This will be done by sticking amended texts over those now superseded. Amending stickers will also be distributed through District Health Promotion Units. In addition the Health Education Authority is promoting the new advice in response to enquiries from press and health professionals.

DR KENNETH CALMAN
Chief Medical Officer

MRS A A B POOLE
Chief Nursing Officer

Current Written Advice from The United Kingdom Health Departments

i) "Back to Sleep" Campaign leaflet

ii) Press advertisement "Back to Sleep"

i) "Back to Sleep" Campaign leaflet

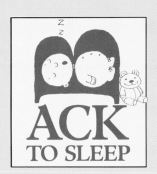

REDUCING

THE RISK OF

COT DEATH

THE DEPARTMENT OF HEALTH

Cot Death, also known as Sudden Infant Death Syndrome, usually affects babies between one and five months. It happens while they're asleep and is always sudden and unexpected. Thankfully, it is comparatively rare.

Because no-one yet knows why Cot Death happens, there's no sure way to prevent it. Studies have shown that by taking a few simple precautions, you can reduce the risk.

The information in this leaflet is for everyone who looks after a baby...not just parents but other members of the family and other carers such as childminders and babysitters.

Why not keep this leaflet next to where your baby sleeps so everyone knows what to do.

● Sleeping Position

Recent research shows that Cot Death is more common in babies who go to sleep on their tummies. By making sure your baby goes to sleep in the right position you can reduce the risk of Cot Death.

Babies should be laid down to sleep:

A) on their backs or,

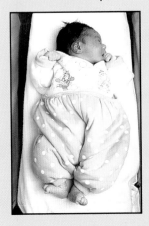

B) on their sides, with the lower arm forward to stop them rolling over.

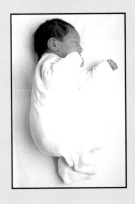
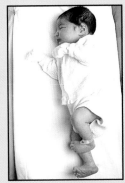

Don't be worried that babies might be sick and choke if laid on their backs. There is no evidence that this happens.

Some babies who require special care or who have particular medical problems need to be nursed on their tummies. Your doctor, nurse or midwife will explain why. If in doubt talk it over with them.

For babies who have been sleeping on their tummies, try them on their backs or sides. But they may not like the change and find it difficult to settle. If this happens then it is probably wise not to upset them by insisting on the new position. If you are at all worried then speak to your health visitor or doctor.

The right sleeping position is only important until babies are able to roll themselves over in their sleep. Once they can do this it is safe to let them take whichever position they prefer.

● Temperature

Babies should be kept warm, but they must not be allowed to get too warm. Keep the temperature in your baby's room so that you feel comfortable in it.

Use lightweight blankets which you can add to or take away according to the room temperature. Do not use a duvet or baby nest which can be too warm and can easily cover a baby's head.

Feverish babies should have few, or even no blankets.

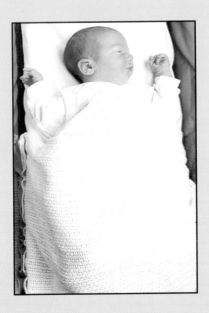

● Smoke-free

Create a smoke-free zone for your baby.
Do not smoke anywhere near the baby.
Better still do not smoke at all.

● **If your baby seems unwell seek
medical advice early and quickly.**

**Research continues into the
causes of Cot Death. Remember
it is comparatively rare, so do not
let the fear of Cot Death spoil the
first months with your baby.**

Further copies of this leaflet are available
by writing to:

> Reducing the Risk of Cot Death
> Health Publications Unit
> No. 2 Site
> Heywood Stores
> Manchester Road
> Heywood
> Lancashire
> OL10 2PZ

ii) Press advertisement "Back to Sleep"

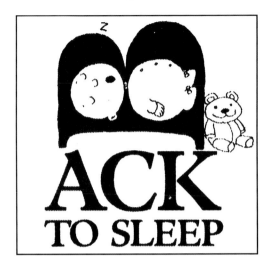

Laying babies to sleep on their back or side greatly reduces the risk of cot death.

Cot death is comparatively rare.

Recent research however, has shown that if babies are laid down to sleep on their back or side the risk of cot death can be greatly reduced.

Don't be worried that they might be sick and choke when on their back. There is no evidence that this happens.

However, there are some babies with special medical problems who need to sleep on their front.

And some babies are used to sleeping on their tummy. Try the new position but if the baby finds it too distressing it is probably wiser not to persist.

If you have any doubts at all, don't hesitate to contact your doctor, midwife or health visitor.

And remember, once babies are strong enough to roll over by themselves, they can sleep in any position they like.

The Department of Health's new leaflet explains in more detail how anyone who looks after a baby can help reduce the risk of cot death.

It's indispensable advice. And if you ask for your copy today, it won't just keep your baby safer, it'll help you sleep more easily too.

Send coupon to The "Back to Sleep" Campaign, FREEPOST, BS 4335, Bristol BSI 3YX. Or phone the leaflet line free any time on 0800 100 160.

Name...

Address...

....

....

....Postcode ....

For your free copy of 'Back to Sleep: Reducing the Risk of Cot Death' fill in the coupon in block capitals and send to The "Back to Sleep" Campaign, FREEPOST BS 4335, Bristol BS1 3YX, or phone the leaflet line free anytime on

0800 100 160.

Sources of Advice from the Health Education Authority

The Health Education Authority (HEA) and the health
education agencies in Scotland, Wales and Northern Ireland
provide a number of booklets which contain information on
infant care. They give specific advice in relation to cot death
and ways of reducing the risks.

The Pregnancy Book

The Pregnancy Book is given free of charge to every first-time
mother. During 1991 revisions were provided, in the form of
stick in slips, to reflect the new advice on the sleeping position
of infants. A new edition of the Pregnancy Book, containing a
much revised account of cot death and advice on reducing the
risk, was published in 1993.

Birth to Five.

This book, which is made available to first-time parents,
contains advice on infant care. During 1991 revisions were
provided, in the form of stick in slips, to reflect the new advice
on the sleeping position of infants. A new edition of the book
was published in December 1992.

Play it Safe!

Play it Safe! is made available to parents of young children. This
leaflet already incorporates the new advice.

Other Relevant Advice from the United Kingdom Health Departments.

Screening for the detection of congenital dislocation of the hip.

In 1986 the Department of Health issued a revision of the handbook "Screening for the detection of congenital dislocation of the hip"[1]. It had been prepared by a Working Party of the Standing Medical Advisory Committee and the Standing Nursing and Midwifery Medical Advisory Committee. In accordance with practice at that time, the handbook contained (at paragraph 2.2) the statement that "new born infants should whenever possible sleep in a prone position". This advice is superseded by the advice on the sleeping position of infants given in this Report.

Reference

1.   Department of Health and Social Security. *Screening for the detection of congenital dislocation of the hip* (Revised 1986). The Standing Medical Advisory Committee and the Standing Nursing and Midwifery Advisory Committee: Department of Health and Social Security, 1986.

What counts as cot Death?

1. There have been discussions and correspondence over what precisely is meant by cot death, sudden infant death, sudden infant death syndrome or similar term,[1,2].

Certification and registration of infant deaths.

2. Different death certificates are used for registering neonatal deaths (those of babies under 28 days) and postneonatal deaths (those of babies aged 28 days and over, up to one year). For postneonatal deaths, as for all deaths at over one year, the certificate allows registrars to record up to three causes of death given by the medical certifier. Following guidelines given by the World Health Organisation's 9th Revision of the International Classification of Diseases (ICD) one term, usually the most precise, is chosen by the Office of Population Censuses and Surveys (OPCS) as the underlying cause of death. Other significant conditions contributing to the death, but not related to the cause of death, may also be entered on the certificate although they are not coded by OPCS. Since 1986, neonatal deaths have been registered differently. In these cases the certifier is able to record **both** main fetal conditions **and** main maternal conditions leading to the death, without giving precedence to one particular condition. Certifiers are also allowed to record other fetal and maternal conditions which contributed to the death although they did not cause it directly. Owing to these changes in the neonatal death certificate it is no longer possible to select a single underlying cause of death for these babies.

3. The following terms which are used by OPCS are variously used in the United Kingdom to describe cot death.

    ### (i) Sudden Infant Death Syndrome - any mention[3,4].

    OPCS Monitor Series DH3, Sudden Infant Death Syndrome (Sudden infant deaths for 1991), records infant deaths for which the death certificate contains any mention of cot death or similar term, such as sudden unexpected infant death, sudden infant death, sudden infant death syndrome. These records include deaths for which other explanations, most commonly respiratory causes, are also given. They include neonatal deaths where in addition to other infant causes there may also be maternal causes. Such certification practice does not accord with the normal use of the term cot death as a diagnosis of exclusion.

(ii) Sudden Infant Death Syndrome - as underlying cause (ICD 9th Revision 798.0)[5].

Deaths assigned to the Sudden Infant Death Syndrome as the underlying cause of death exclude those deaths where mention is made of any (other) definitive cause. The rules by which such assignments are made are laid down by WHO. Statistics on this basis are published in OPCS Annual Reference Volume Series DH6: Mortality statistics: childhood.

(iii) Sudden Death - cause unknown (ICD 798)[5].

When used in respect of deaths during infancy and early childhood, this underlying cause category contains a few events other than those assigned to the Sudden Infant Death Syndrome. It does, however, encompass a small number of deaths of unknown cause of 'abandoned ' babies.

(iv) Signs, symptoms and ill-defined conditions (ICD 780-799)[6].

Under the age of 1 year the majority of deaths assigned to this somewhat broader underlying cause category are attributed to the Sudden Infant Death Syndrome. It may be that, with the exception of those associated with abandonment, the remainder may not differ from cot deaths.

4.   It has been remarked[2] that for cot deaths which occur during the postneonatal period, the figures described at paragraphs 3ii - iv are virtually the same.

5.   Different studies have used different case definitions of cot death. Some have included neonatal deaths, some only postperinatal deaths (deaths after 7 days), and some have included deaths beyond the first year. However, all studies have included postneonatal deaths, among which over 90% of cot

deaths are to be found.

6. Studies have also differed in the proportion of deaths attributed to cot death in which there was a full investigation, including postmortem examination; and in those deaths which were the subject of postmortem examination there were variations in the depth and scope of investigation.

7. We are confident that such differences between studies which have been the sources of our evidence do not threaten our conclusions or the recommendations derived from them.

References

1. Limerick SR, Gardner A. What counts as cot death? *BMJ* 1992; 304: 1176.

2. Gordon RR. What counts as cot death? *BMJ* 1992; 304: 1508.

3. Office of Population Censuses and Surveys. *Sudden infant deaths*. OPCS monitor series DH3. London: HMSO, 1980-1990. (DH3 80/3 to 91/1).

4. Office of Population Censuses and Surveys. *Sudden infant death syndrome*. OPCS monitor series DH3, London: HMSO, 1980-90. (DH3 92/2).

5. Office of Population Censuses and Surveys. *Mortality statistics: childhood*. Annual Reference Volume Series DH6. London: HMSO, 1986-91 (DH6 1-5).

6. Office of Population Censuses and Surveys. *Cause of death XVI signs, symptoms and ill-defined conditions*. ICD 780-799. 20 days to 1 year., VS3 series. London: HMSO, 1986-90.

OPCS Ominbus Surveys of public awareness of 'Back to Sleep'.

Each month, interviews are conducted with approximately 2,000 adult individuals (aged 16 or over) in private households in Great Britain. The sampling frame is the Postcode Address File of "small users", which includes all private household addresses. A new sample of 100 postal sectors is selected for each month, with stratification by region, the proportion of households renting from local authorities, and the proportion in which the head of household is in Socio-Economic Groups 1-5 or 13 (ie a professional, employer or manager). The postal sectors are selected with probability proportionate to size and, within each sector, 30 addresses are selected randomly.

If an address contains more than one household, the interviewer uses a standard OPCS procedure to select just one household randomly. Within households with more than one adult member, just one person aged 16 or over is selected with the use of random number tables. The interviewer endeavours to interview that person and no proxies are taken.

Because only one household member is interviewed, people in households containing few adults have a better change of selection than those in households with many. A weighting factor is applied to correct for this.

This survey was used in March and November to assess public awareness of the messages of the "Back to Sleep" campaign, in the aftermath and subsequently.

Table 1 summarises the responses obtained from a sample of 1365 individuals, during March 1992, to the following question and subsequent probing:

Thinking about everything you have heard or seen recently about reducing the risk of cot death, what advice has been given? (Probe: Anything else?)

RECORD ANSWERS VERBATIM THEN CODE BELOW (CODE ALL THAT APPLY, INCL. 'OTHER')

Put baby to sleep on back or side, not front..

Put baby to sleep on front, not back or side...

Advice about position of baby, unspecified...

Don't let baby get too hot, don't cover with too many blankets ....

Don't allow cigarette smoke near baby/don't smoke in same room.....................

Other..

Table 2 summarises the responses obtained from a sample of 1521 individuals, during November 1992, to the following questions and subsequent probing:

What do you know about reducing the risk of cot death?
(Probe: Anything else?)

RECORD ANSWERS VERBATIM THEN CODE BELOW (CODE ALL THAT APPLY, INCL 'OTHER').

Put baby to sleep on back or side, not front...

Put baby to sleep on front, not back or side...

Vaguer about position of baby...

Don't let baby get to hot, don't cover with too many blankets................................

Don't allow cigarette smoke near baby/don't smoke in same room........................

Avoid smoking while pregnant ....

Some other advice mentioned..

Not interested/not relevant (children too old/no children etc)...............................

Don't remember/don't know ....

In March 1992, among women in child-bearing age groups (16-24, 25-44 years), 82 and 86% were aware of the advice to put a baby to sleep on its back or its side, not the front; 48 and 50% were aware of advice not to let a baby get too hot; and 13 and 15% were aware of advice not to expose a baby to cigarette smoke. In November 1992 the respective figures were 60 and 77%; 50 and 62%; and 13 and 20%.

The majority among these groups of women were aware of the message on the sleeping position of babies. but it must be reinforced. The message on the risks of overheating was known by about half of them and should be known more widely. The message on exposing a baby to cigarette smoke was the least well known.

In March 1992, among women in child-bearing age groups (16-24, 25-44 years) 73 and 87% had heard or seen the message on reducing the risks: from television 82 and 87%; from newspapers or magazine 36 and 45%; from health professionals 12 and 6%; from the Department of Health leaflet 20 and 13%; and privately 5 and 5%. In November 1992, 78 and 86% had heard or seen the message on reducing the risks: from television 88 and 86%; from newspapers or magazine 41 and 61%; from health professionals 18 and 27%; from the Department of Health leaflet 18 and 22%; and privately 15 and 18%.

During the period March - November 1992 increasing numbers of women in these groups heard messages on reducing the risk of cot death from health professionals and through private conversation. This suggests that the new advice on reducing the risks of cot death is becoming an accepted part of health professional practice and public culture.

Further surveys are planned

Table 1. Responses from a sample of 1365 individuals during March 1992 to the question (with probing): "Thinking about everything you have heard or seen recently about reducing the risk of cot deaths, what advise has been given?

*Question with subsequent probing	Male							Female						
	Age						Total	Age						Total
	16 to 24	25 to 44	45 to 54	55 to 64	65 to 74	75 and over		16 to 24	25 to 44	45 to 54	55 to 64	65 to 74	75 and over	
What advice given														
Put baby on back/side....	36	160	61	60	45	18	380	95	281	100	102	59	31	668
	55%	68%	66%	74%	65%	73%	67%	82%	86%	85%	82%	79%	79%	84%
Put baby on front....	6	9	5	4	7	0	31	3	12	2	1	1	1	20
	9%	4%	6%	4%	10%	0%	5%	3%	4%	2%	1%	1%	1%	2%
Advice - position unspecified....	8	23	3	8	4	0	46	8	14	5	8	5	1	40
	12%	10%	3%	9%	5%	0%	8%	7%	4%	4%	7%	6%	3%	5%
Not get too hot....	12	65	12	17	13	3	122	58	156	40	40	20	8	322
	18%	28%	13%	21%	18%	12%	22%	50%	48%	34%	32%	27%	21%	40%
Not smoke, no smoke in room	6	17	1	3	0	0	27	18	41	11	6	0	0	76
	9%	7%	1%	4%	0%	0%	5%	15%	13%	10%	5%	0%	0%	10%
Other....	32	91	42	36	23	10	234	37	108	39	36	24	9	254
	49%	39%	46%	44%	33%	42%	41%	32%	33%	33%	29%	33%	23%	32%
Base....	66	235	92	81	69	24	567	115	327	117	124	75	39	798
	100%	100%	100%	100%	100%	100%	100%	100%	100%	100%	100%	100%	100%	100%

*. See text for details

105

Table 2. Responses from a sample of 1521 individuals during November 1992 to the question (with probing): "What do you know about reducing the risk of cot death?"

*Question with subsequent probing	Male							Female						
	Age						Total	Age						Total
	16 to 24	25 to 44	45 to 54	55 to 64	65 to 74	75 and over		16 to 24	25 to 44	45 to 54	55 to 64	65 to 74	75 and over	
Know to reduce risks?														
Put baby on back/side....	32 / 42%	133 / 55%	62 / 59%	50 / 55%	49 / 60%	25 / 58%	351 / 55%	66 / 60%	266 / 77%	113 / 82%	103 / 80%	76 / 73%	31 / 57%	655 / 74%
Put baby on front....	6 / 8%	31 / 13%	5 / 5%	2 / 2%	6 / 8%	3 / 7%	54 / 8%	11 / 10%	20 / 6%	5 / 4%	4 / 3%	3 / 3%	1 / 2%	44 / 5%
Advice - position unspecified....	19 / 25%	26 / 11%	8 / 8%	12 / 13%	4 / 5%	0 / 0%	69 / 11%	17 / 15%	25 / 7%	14 / 10%	10 / 8%	3 / 3%	3 / 5%	72 / 8%
Not get too hot....	9 / 12%	71 / 29%	15 / 14%	19 / 21%	10 / 13%	3 / 7%	126 / 20%	55 / 50%	216 / 62%	68 / 49%	56 / 44%	29 / 28%	11 / 21%	436 / 49%
Not smoke, no smoke in room....	5 / 6%	19 / 8%	1 / 1%	4 / 4%	3 / 4%	0 / 0%	32 / 5%	15 / 13%	70 / 20%	17 / 12%	6 / 4%	5 / 5%	0 / 0%	111 / 13%
Avoid smoking while pregnant....	1 / 1%	4 / 2%	0 / 0%	1 / 1%	1 / 1%	1 / 1%	6 / 1%	5 / 5%	26 / 7%	5 / 3%	6 / 4%	1 / 1%	0 / 0%	43 / 5%
Some advice mentioned....	25 / 34%	78 / 32%	27 / 25%	16 / 18%	26 / 31%	5 / 12%	177 / 28%	34 / 31%	117 / 34%	45 / 33%	34 / 27%	23 / 23%	14 / 26%	268 / 30%
Not interested/not relevant....	7 / 9%	30 / 12%	24 / 23%	22 / 25%	15 / 18%	15 / 35%	113 / 18%	6 / 5%	17 / 5%	8 / 6%	11 / 9%	19 / 18%	16 / 29%	77 / 9%
Base....	75 / 100%	243 / 100%	104 / 100%	90 / 100%	83 / 100%	44 / 100%	639 / 100%	111 / 100%	347 / 100%	138 / 100%	129 / 100%	103 / 100%	54 / 100%	882 / 100%

*See text for details

Sleeping Position of Infants Studies in Avon and Isle of Man, UK

Data on the sleeping position of infants, preceding and following the national campaign, has been provided by Professor Jean Golding and Dr Peter Fleming. The data came from the Avon Longitudinal Study of Pregnancy and Childhood (ALSPAC), and includes over 80% of births in the three Bristol-based health districts of Avon, UK.

When their baby was 4-8 weeks of age, mothers were asked the position in which their baby was laid to sleep at night, and the position in which the baby was found in the morning. The self-completion questionnaires allowed the options: back, front, side, and "varies". Table 1 gives the percentage of babies for whom a clear preference had been stated for laying down, ie omitting 2-4% described as "varies". The percentage placed on their fronts declined until the beginning of October 1991, and then there was a fall towards the end of October so that during November and December the percentage of babies laid on their fronts fell to 1%. It remained at 3% or less until June 1992 when the latest data were made available. The percentage of babies laid on their backs gradually increased from 5% during September to 27% by January and 40% by June 1992. This was accompanied by a fall in the percentage of babies placed on their side.

Data on the wakening position shows that the percentage of babies awakening on their fronts fell to 2% in November 1991 and remained at this level thereafter. This suggests that babies who are placed on their sides were placed in such a way that they did not roll onto their front, but rather onto their backs. The percentage awakening on their backs did not change until January 1992, when it increased to 57%, with a further increase to 76% in May and June.

Conclusion

In Avon a local publicity campaign aimed at changing sleeping position had begun in 1990-91. The data given in Table 1 suggest that the national campaign from November 1991 had an immediate and profound effect on the sleeping position of infants in this population.

Data are also available from mothers taking part in the European Longitudinal Study of Pregnancy and Childhood (ELSPAC) who live on the

Isle of Man. ALSPAC is a contributor to this study also and similar methods are used. Practice in respect of infant sleeping position can therefore be compared in these two areas. Table 2 shows the position of infants on being laid down to sleep and on awakening during the period January - October 1991. The results obtained before the national campaign in November 1991, were almost identical in the two areas. No campaign had been conducted on the Isle of Man. These findings suggest that the sleeping position of babies may have been changing throughout the British Isles even though no overt targeted campaign had taken place[1].

Further data are expected from the ELSPAC and ALSPAC studies.

1. Golding J, Fleming PJ, Parkes S. Cot deaths and sleeping position campaigns. *Lancet* 1992; 339: 748-9.

Table 1. **Position of infants, aged 4-8 weeks, when laid down to sleep and on awakening. September 1991 - June 1992 Avon, UK.**

Month	When Laid Down			On Awakening		
			Percentage (numbers)			
	Back	Front	Side	Back	Front	Side
Sept 1991	5% (26)	10% (59)	85% (493)	40% (203)	12% (61)	48% (239)
Oct 1991	6% (36)	7% (43)	87% (535)	31% (172)	8% (45)	61% (337)
Nov 1991	13% (115)	2% (15)	85% (778)	40% (349)	2% (13)	58% (503)
Dec 1991	23% (195)	1% (9)	76% (651)	49% (369)	2% (11)	49% (370)
Jan 1992	27% (295)	3% (35)	70% (760)	57% (599)	3% (27)	60% (626)
Feb 1992	30% (182)	2% (12)	68% (417)	60% (348)	2% (11)	38% (224)
Mar 1992	31% (173)	1% (7)	68% (382)	57% (358)	2% (11)	41% (258)
Apr 1992	29% (59)	5% (1)	70% (143)	54% (105)	2% (3)	44% (85)
May 1992	38% (243)	6% (4)	61% (395)	76% (476)	1% (5)	23% (143)
June 1992	40% (198)	2% (10)	58% (284)	76% (369)	2% (11)	22% (103)

Unpubished data: Professor Jean Golding

Table 2. **Position of infants, aged 4-8 weeks, when laid down to sleep and on awakening. January - October 1991, Avon and Isle of Man, UK.**

	When Laid Down		On Awakening	
	Avon	Isle of Man	Avon	Isle of Man
Position	(n=1120)	(n=403)	(n=1120)	(n=400)
Back	2% (27)	4% (16)	26% (286)	28% (117)
Side	78% (868)	75% (301)	40% (450)	33% (131)
Front	14% (159)	16% (65)	14% (160)	15% (59)
Varies	6% (66)	5% (21)	20% (224)	23% (92)

Glossary

(Terms in *italics* appear in the Glossary also).

Aetiology, aetiological

Relating to the causes of disease in populations. Aetiological studies aim to discover

(i) the overall incidence of diseases or categories of death in a population, and

(ii) what factors determine which particular individuals within a population fall sick or die.

Case-control (see also: *cohort*)

Case control studies compare the subjects who experience a particular outcome with those – *controls*, or comparison groups – who do not. Such studies are also described as *retrospective*, in that they look back to suspected causes. The means of selecting controls to ensure as far as possible that the differences between them and cases reflect exposure to the suspected causes - and not to *confounding factors* – is a critical aspect of such studies. Many are flawed because of their failure to take confounding factors into account.

Causal

A factor which is strongly associated with a particular outcome is not necessarily a cause of that outcome. The association might have occurred by chance; or it might simply reflect an association with some other factor which is itself causally related to the outcome (a *confounding factor*).

Cohort (see also: *case -control*)

Cohort studies compare a particular outcome in subjects who are exposed to a particular factor with subjects who are not – *controls*. They are also called *prospective* studies.

Confounding factor or variable

A factor that is associated with a suspected *risk factor* for a particular outcome, and which independently determines the risk of that outcome. For example, the likelihood of not breast feeding is strongly associated with maternal smoking. Maternal smoking is strongly associated with cot death; therefore in studies to determine the association between not breast feeding

110

and cot death, maternal smoking is a confounding variable and must be taken into account in the analysis.

Congenital anomaly

A physical malformation which is present at birth.

Control (see: *case-control, cohort*)

Epidemiology

The study of the distribution and determinants of disease and death in human populations.

Festschrift (ger. Fest, Festival: schrift, writings).

A tribute to a scholar, in the form of papers, essays etc, on some special occasion (usually on retirement or a particular anniversary).

Frequency (see also: *incidence, prevalence*).

A term used to describe the number of events (cases) in a specified period, often without reference to the populations at risk.

Gastro-oesophageal reflux

The state of affairs when stomach contents return silently to the throat, often during sleep, from which they might enter the lungs. This is potentially harmful.

Incidence (see also: *frequency, prevalence*)

Incidence rate is the number of events in relation to numbers in a defined population and a specified period.

Infant (see also: *mortality rate*)

There are several usages. In the UK it means a child in the first year of life.

Intervention study

An experimental study in a defined population in which a suspected *aetiological* factor is changed and the consequences are assessed. For example, changes in the incidence of cot death have been determined following changes in the sleeping position of infants.

Matched (see also: *case-control, cohort*).

In *aetiological* studies the selection of study and control subjects must ensure that, as far as knowledge of the disorder allows, the two groups of subjects are equally susceptible, and are therefore matched in respect of *confounding variables*.

Mortality rate

In this Report the following mortality rates are used:

Infant mortality rate.
The number of *infants* who die during a stated year per 1,000 live births occurring in the same year.

Neonatal mortality rate.
The number of infants who die in the *neonatal* period during a stated year per 1,000 live births occurring in the same year.

Postneonatal mortality rate.
The number of infants who die in the *postneonatal* period during a stated year per 1,000 live births occurring in the same year.

Neonatal (see also: *infant, postneonatal*)
Refers to events in the first 28 days of life.

Odds ratio

A statistical term which quantifies the likelihood of a given outcome in those exposed to an aetiological factor compared with those who are not.

Pierre-Robin Syndrome

A congenital disorder characterised by an underdeveloped lower jaw, a poorly anchored tongue, which is displaced backwards and downwards, and a high-arched, often cleft palate. The clinical features are due to respiratory obstruction and difficulty in swallowing. Distress is worse in the supine position or when feeding.

Postneonatal (see also: *infant, neonatal*)
Refers to events after the first 28 days of life, up to the end of the first year.

Prevalence (see also: *incidence*)
Prevalence describes the proportion of people in a specified population who are affected by a disorder at one particular time.

Prospective (see: *cohort*)

Relative risk (see also: *risk factor*)

An expression of the strength of a suspected *risk factor* for a particular outcome. It is the ratio of the *incidence* of the outcome in those exposed to the incidence in those who are not.

Retrospective (see : *case-control*)

Risk factor (see also: *relative risk*)

A health hazard to individuals who are exposed.

Significance, significant

In statistics relates to the difference in outcome observed between study and control groups. Such a difference might be due to faulty design or conduct of the study. But it might be due to chance, in which case statistical significance should be calculated to take into account this possible explanation.

Unmatched (see: *matched*)

Printed in the United Kingdom for HMSO

Dd 296391, C15.7, 6/93